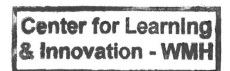

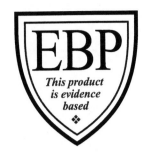

EBP

This product is evidence based

Evidence-Based Staff Development

Strategies to Create, Measure, and Refine Your Program

Adrianne E. Avillion, DEd, RN

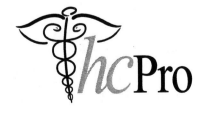

*hc*Pro

Evidence-Based Staff Development: Strategies to Create, Measure, and Refine Your Program is published by HCPro, Inc.

ISBN 978-1-60146-039-4

Adrianne E. Avillion, DEd, RN, Author
Rebecca Hendren, Managing Editor
Lindsey Cardarelli, Associate Editor
Emily Sheahan, Group Publisher
Shane Katz, Cover Designer
Jackie Diehl Singer, Graphic Artist
Genevieve d'Entremont, Copyeditor

Sada Preisch, Proofreader
Darren Kelly, Books Production Supervisor
Susan Darbyshire, Art Director
Claire Cloutier, Production Manager
Jean St. Pierre, Director of Operations
Paul Singer, Layout Artist

Arrangements can be made for quantity discounts. For more information, contact:

HCPro, Inc.
P.O. Box 1168
Marblehead, MA 01945
Telephone: 800/650-6787 or 781/639-1872
Fax: 781/639-2982
E-mail: *customerservice@hcpro.com*

Visit HCPro at its World Wide Web sites:
www.hcpro.com and *www.hcmarketplace.com*

Contents

About the author

Adrianne E. Avillion, DEd, RN

Adrianne E. Avillion, DEd, RN, is the owner of Avillion's Curriculum Design in York, PA. A past president of the National Nursing Staff Development Organization (NNSDO), she specializes in freelance medical writing and designing continuing education programs for healthcare professionals. She also offers consulting services in the areas of work redesign, quality improvement, and staff development.

Avillion has published extensively and has served as editor of the first and second editions of *The Core Curriculum for Staff Development*, published by NNSDO. Her most recent publications include *A Practical Guide to Staff Development: Tools and Techniques for Effective Education*, published by HCPro, Inc., and *Nurse Entrepreneurship: The Art of Running Your Own Business*, published by Creative Health Care Management in Minneapolis, MN. She is also a frequent presenter at conferences and conventions devoted to the specialty of continuing education and staff development.

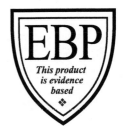

EBP

This product is evidence based

Purpose and rationale for evidence-based staff development practice

Purpose and rationale for evidence-based staff development practice

Learning objective

After reading this chapter, the participant will be able to:

• Explain the use of evidence in staff development practice

Introduction

Evidence-based practice (EBP) is a hot topic among healthcare professionals. EBP is the process of making clinical decisions based on the most current and valid research and highest-quality data available, with the goal of improving patient safety and decreasing the number of medical errors (Krugman 2003). Staff development specialists are often called upon to teach the concepts of EBP and to act as facilitators of its implementation. This is neither surprising nor unusual, since staff development specialists are viewed as innovators who play key roles in organizational change.

But what about EBP's application in our own practice setting, the specialty of staff development? Even as we help our colleagues implement EBP in clinical settings, our own practice is in critical need of similar evidence-based strategies. If the rationale for clinical EBP is its positive impact on patient outcomes and patient safety, the rationale for staff development EBP must be similar. When employees receive better training and continuing education, they are better able to do their jobs. It is presumed that enhanced job performance leads to better patient care and improved patient outcomes.

The purpose of this book is to help staff development specialists improve the effectiveness of their products and services through the implementation of evidence-based practice. Such implementation involves an analysis of EBP as it pertains to staff development, evaluation of current practice, and identification of strategies for the successful implementation of EBP in the staff development setting.

Are we ready to implement EBP in our staff development work? We should be, based on the evolution of the specialty and the role we play in our work settings. But there are some serious obstacles to the implementation of EBP in staff development that we must work to eliminate.

The two primary obstacles to implementation are the lack of credible staff development research and, practically speaking, insufficient understanding of the concept as it relates to the specialty. Some of us are still struggling with the assessment of application, impact on organizational effectiveness, and return on investment (ROI) of our services. We need to be able to successfully conduct the evaluation process and utilize its findings (and those of other research studies) to properly implement EBP in staff development.

EBP TIP *Remember, a properly conducted evaluation is also research! Don't make the mistake of thinking research must be conducted by doctorally prepared individuals, take months or even years to complete, and be so statistically complex that it is almost incomprehensible to most staff development specialists. You have probably conducted (and are continuing to conduct) more research studies than you know. The trick is to recognize research and findings, and figure out how to apply them. This is the essence of evidence-based staff development practice.*

Evidence as a road map for staff development: Using Benner's work as an example

Many staff development specialists are familiar with the work of Patricia Benner (1984). Her descriptive research, based on dialogues with nurses with various levels of clinical expertise, identified five levels of competency in clinical nursing. These levels are not based on passage of time or the number of years participants had been registered nurses; instead, they are based on an analysis of the data collected. As an example of using research findings to guide practice, let's look at Benner's five levels of clinical experience and determine if they could be applied to staff development specialists.

EBP TIP *Use this example as a way to think about other available data that may be used to implement evidence-based staff development practice. Let your imagination explore the possibilities.*

Level 1: Novice

Novices are beginning practitioners with no experience of the situations in which they are expected to perform (Benner 1984). Clinically, novices are nursing students or nurses who have no experience working with a particular patient population. Likewise, novices may be registered nurses with years of clinical experience, but none in staff development. Consider this scenario.

Marlene is a registered nurse with 10 years of clinical experience. Her specialty is women's oncology. She is known for her efforts to help less experienced colleagues learn about the intricacies of oncology nursing. However, Marlene has had no formal education or continuing education pertaining to staff development. She tells Angela, the director of the staff development department, that she would like to pursue a career in this specialty. Angela knows that teaching experience is a prerequisite for employment in her department. Therefore, Marlene needs some instruction in the teaching/learning process. How will Angela use evidence-based data to help Marlene?

If you were in Angela's place, what would you do first, based on your background in staff development? In other words, what does the data you've collected from years of experience tell you to do? Angela may encourage Marlene to pursue both formal and continuing education opportunities in the staff development field. She may also begin to include Marlene in developing and presenting specific inservices and/or continuing education offerings on the oncology unit.

Experience tells you that Marlene needs rules to guide her performance. Data tells you that there are certain fundamentals of education that need to be understood and applied in order to develop a successful learning activity. Rules to guide Marlene include:

- Principles of adult learning
- Education process (needs assessment, planning, implementation, and evaluation)
- Writing objectives

Obviously there is much more to becoming a successful staff development specialist than these initial guidelines. But Marlene needs these basic rules as a foundation for practice.

You may not have conducted formal research concerning Marlene's initial instruction, but you know from educational literature and experience that these guidelines are essential as starting points. Evidence tells you that without an understanding of these basics, Marlene will not be able to progress to the next level of expertise. At this level, Marlene is not able to perform any of the tasks these guidelines require; she is depending on you to teach her how to function within the parameters set by these basic rules.

Level 2: Advanced beginner

Advanced beginners are those nurses who "can demonstrate marginally acceptable performance, ones who have coped with enough real situations to note (or to have pointed out to them by a mentor) the recurring meaningful situational components that are termed 'aspects of the situation'" (Benner 1984). Advanced beginners have enough prior experience to perform some aspects of planning, implementation, and evaluation. However, these aspects are ones with which they have had prior experience.

Advanced beginners are not sure how to handle new situations (e.g., encountering resistant learners or content that does not meet learner needs, requiring "on-the-spot" changes). Like novices, they need guidelines to deal with unfamiliar or unexpected situations as well as guidance in how to prioritize tasks. They treat all challenges as equally important.

 EVIDENCE-BASED STAFF DEVELOPMENT

Daniel has worked in the staff development department for about one year. His clinical background as an emergency department nurse allows him to concentrate on critical care aspects of continuing education. Recently, he planned and implemented a continuing education program that consisted of a lecture/discussion component as well as a skill return demonstration. This was the first time Daniel completed this type of activity (from start to finish) without assistance from more experienced staff development colleagues. Program evaluations were quite good, with 40 out of 50 participants rating the instructor, teaching methods, and achievement of objectives as very good to excellent. Five participants rated the program as below average, stating that the return demonstration component took too long to complete and that it was difficult to leave the work setting to attend. Five participants rated the program as poor, the major complaints being that the lecture/discussion component allowed insufficient time to achieve objectives, and that Daniel did not allow enough time for questions and discussion.

Daniel, in an attempt to follow evaluation guidelines that require using participant feedback to revise programs as necessary, begins an elaborate revision of his program. He plans to meet with the five participants who rated the program as poor, and begins to revise time frames and objectives. As an advanced beginner, Daniel is following guidelines, and treating all data obtained as equally important.

Based on evidence, how would you help Daniel?

A more experienced staff development specialist would not have a "knee-jerk" reaction to the 10 negative comments. You should help Daniel to look at all the data before planning any action. This is not to say that the 10 dissatisfied participants' comments should be discounted because there are so few of them; instead, Daniel needs to look at more than just reactions. For example, in addition to reaction data, how well did participants perform on any posttests and the required skill demonstration? This indicates both knowledge acquisition and skill competency in a controlled situation. Are participants satisfactorily applying new knowledge and skills in the actual work setting?

Analysis of these types of data allows Daniel to make a more accurate assessment of the effectiveness (or lack of effectiveness) of his program. He may wish to make discussion more prominent in the lecture/discussion component of the program and look at time frames. What he should not do is begin revisions without looking at all of the available evidence and prioritizing any necessary alterations.

Daniel is relying on evidence obtained from evaluation data. However, he lacks the experience to analyze findings and prioritize their implications. Yes, Daniel is relying on evidence, but he is not conducting a thorough analysis, nor is he prioritizing appropriately.

Level 3: Competent

The competent nurse has worked in the same or similar circumstances for between two and three years. Competency is characterized by an individual's ability to correlate actions with long-range goals (Benner 1984). A competent staff development specialist is able to deal with many of the complexities of education delivery and is aware of consciously and deliberately planning actions. However, he or she lacks the speed and efficiency of a proficient practitioner.

The necessity to change plans swiftly and/or unexpectedly, and dealing with unanticipated problems (e.g., disruptive learners, administrative demands, or abrupt schedule changes), are quite challenging to the competent staff development specialist.

Laura has worked as a staff development specialist for three years in a large three-hospital health system. Her primary areas of responsibility include implementation of certified nursing assistant programs and inservice and continuing education for the 200-bed neurologic rehabilitation center. Many of the registered nurses who work in the rehabilitation center hold certifications in rehabilitation and neurological nursing, and they rely on Laura to provide cutting-edge continuing education. These nurses are finding it increasingly difficult to leave their work settings to attend classroom-style programs. However, their written and verbal feedback data indicate their resistance to distance learning and preference for "in-person" programs during which they can interact and participate in question-and-answer sessions.

As a result of accrediting agency surveyor recommendations and organizational goals, Laura is told to revise as many programs as possible to a distance learning format. Laura is adamantly opposed to this idea. She believes that distance learning could not be as effective as classroom interaction for the various programs she must implement. She tells her manager that she is going to use evidence from program evaluations as well as the results of assessing knowledge acquisition and application in the work setting to justify offering programs in their current format.

If you were Laura's manager, what would you do?

It is the way evidence is used, rather than the evidence itself, that is the issue in this scenario. Laura lacks the flexibility and efficiency of the proficient nurse. You should help Laura look at this situation objectively. The evidence shows that:

© 2007 HCPro, Inc. **EVIDENCE-BASED STAFF DEVELOPMENT**

- Participants have expressed a preference for classroom-style learning, where they can interact and discuss issues

- Attendance at such programs is declining and nurses have expressed concern that it is difficult to leave their respective work areas to attend these programs

- Participants have acquired knowledge and successfully applied new knowledge in the actual work setting

- Accrediting agency surveyors have suggested incorporating distance learning into Laura's programs

- Administrative mandates include the incorporation of distance learning

Although Laura should not automatically convert all programs in their entirety to a distance learning format, evidence indicates that she needs to consider the incorporation of distance learning when it will enhance educational outcomes.

Start by analyzing each program. With the help of her manager, Laura should identify which programs could be suitably reformatted for distance learning, and should remember that blended learning methodologies (e.g., a self-learning module and a skill demonstration) are often very successful.

Laura could start with the program that seems most adaptable and pilot it on certain groups of nurses. More evidence or data will then be collected and used to continue her evaluation of the feasibility of distance learning. Laura needs to increase her flexibility and her ability to objectively analyze data and use evidence to meet the needs of all of her customers, including members of the administrative team. Laura's attempt to use evidence to resist surveyors' and administration's recommendations is unwise, both educationally and politically.

Level 4: Proficient

Proficiency is characterized by an almost instinctive perception of a situation as a whole, rather than as individual aspects. A proficient nurse knows what to expect in various staff development situations and how to revise plans in response to changes in such situations (Benner 1984).

Greta is the manager of a staff development department in a large metropolitan health system. She has over 15 years of staff development and management experience. Greta was hired for her present position only six weeks ago. She was employed to redesign delivery of staff development services throughout the health system. In this capacity, she will function as a change agent as well as staff development manager.

How will Greta rely on available evidence to begin her work?

Greta has a huge task in front of her. She will collect both objective data (e.g., from performance evaluations, program evaluations, risk management and quality improvement reports) and subjective data (e.g., meeting with her staff, managers throughout the health system, administrative staff, and members of the clinical and nonclinical staff). Data analysis must include accreditation survey results, as well as the quality and appropriateness of educational programming.

As a proficient staff development specialist, Greta knows how to absorb the "big picture," prioritize needs, and make long-range plans. She has learned from experience what may and may not work and how to anticipate both successes and challenges.

Level 5: Expert

The expert nurse does not rely on rules or guidelines to understand a situation and take effective action; instead, he or she intuitively operates from a complex understanding of a total situation. The expert may have difficulty explaining why a particular decision was made or action taken, simply saying, "It just feels right" (Benner 1984).

The expert staff development specialist is experienced, flexible, and extremely proficient. He or she can swiftly plan, implement, and revise programming with ease and produce successful outcomes.

Ellen is an expert staff development specialist. She finds that she is feeling bored and restless, complaining that "there just isn't anything challenging to do anymore." Ellen is concerned about the lack of valid and reliable staff development evidence to help guide the specialty as a whole and her colleagues as individuals.

What might Ellen do to expand her significant expertise?

Ellen is in an excellent position to add to the body of knowledge that is staff development. Valid and reliable evidence depends on the accurate description of events and on carefully developed research investigations.

However, the expert staff development specialist faces and poses some significant challenges. Less experienced staff development specialists turn to the expert for advice and opinions. The expert may be asked to assume more responsibilities based on her or his expertise and competency. This can cause the expert to experience burnout and frustration.

The expert staff development specialist may become easily bored and believe that new, exciting opportunities are no longer available. It is up to all of us to help experts add to their knowledge bases and pursue new challenges. Such challenges may include spearheading staff development research projects, pursuing additional graduate or postgraduate education, or assuming responsibility for projects at the upper management level. It is unacceptable to lose the experts in our specialty to boredom or burnout.

As you begin to plan for EBP in staff development, you may find it helpful to determine the level of expertise of each of the staff development specialists in your department. (Don't forget to include yourself in this evaluation.) Figure 1.1 offers a template for just such an assessment.

1.1 **Staff development specialist levels of expertise**

Level	Characteristics	Interventions	Comments

Novice	• Beginning practitioner
	
	• No experience of the situations in which he or she is expected to perform
		• Provide rules to guide their performance
		
		• Provide education opportunities in the field of staff development
		
		• Offer instruction concerning:
		
		  - Principles of adult learning
		  - Education process
		  - Writing objectives	

Advanced beginner	• Demonstrates marginally acceptable performance • Has coped with enough "real life" situations to identify recurring meaningful components • Can perform some aspects of program planning, implementation, and evaluation • Is not sure how to handle new situations • Treats all challenges as equally important	• Provide guidelines for dealing with unfamiliar or unexpected situations • Provide guidelines regarding task prioritization • Provide practice scenarios or case studies that allow data analysis and formulating a plan of action	
Competent	• Has worked in the same or similar circumstances for 2–3 years • Correlates actions with long-range goals • Can deal with complex challenges	• Explain strategies to deal with unexpected program demands • Offer options to implement swift, on-the-spot program revision • Provide case studies or other	

Figure 1.1   **Staff development specialist levels of expertise (cont.)**

Level	Characteristics	Interventions	Comments
	• Plans actions consciously and deliberately • Lacks speed and efficiency of proficient staff development specialists	scenarios that help the competent specialist to increase speed and efficiency	
Proficient	• Displays an almost instinctive perception of a situation as a whole rather than individual aspects • Can anticipate challenges that occur in various staff development situations • Can revise plans in response to on-the-spot changes in such situations • Can make long-range plans and prioritize needs	• Offer opportunities to assume some aspects of managerial responsibilities • Offer opportunities to participate in essential committees such as ANCC Magnet Recognition Program® status and Quality Improvement • Facilitate perusal of graduate education and/or management training	
Expert	• Does not need rules or guidelines • Performs intuitively • Swiftly grasps the complexity of a situation and takes immediate action to correct or improve situations as needed • May become bored and unable to identify new opportunities • May become burned out as less experienced staff development specialists turn to her or him for help and advice	• Recognize signs of burnout and frustration and intervene • Offer opportunities to assume responsibility for projects at the upper management level • Facilitate pursuit of graduate or postgraduate education • Offer opportunities to spearhead staff development research projects	

The purpose of this book is to offer you a road map for the development and implementation of evidence-based staff development, as well as to encourage endeavors in staff development research. Staff development specialists are often called upon to help clinicians conduct research investigations and use resulting data to improve patient outcomes. It is time that we called upon ourselves to conduct research specific to staff development and use these findings to improve our own practice.

References

Benner, P. (1984). *From Novice to Expert: Excellence and Power in Clinical Nursing Practice.* Menlo Park, CA: Addison-Wesley.

Krugman, M. (2003). "Evidence-based practice: The role of staff development." *Journal for Nurses in Staff Development*, 19(6), 279–285.

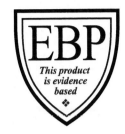

EBP
*This product
is evidence
based*

Overview of the
evidence-based
practice movement

Overview of the evidence-based practice movement

Learning objectives

After reading this chapter, the participant will be able to:

- Review sources for gathering data/evidence for staff development practice
- Summarize the historical issues that contribute to evidence-based staff development practice

Explanation of terms

It is important to differentiate between evidence-based clinical practice and evidence-based staff development practice. The concept of evidence is obviously critical to both. However, some healthcare professionals may believe that evidence-based practice (EBP) is only valid in clinical situations.

EBP is appropriate to any setting. It implies that the effectiveness of a department is continually assessed and that such assessment leads to ongoing efforts to improve products and services.

Evidence-based clinical practice

EBP involves a continual analysis of healthcare practices for the identification and implementation of patient interventions that improve the quality and appropriateness of care. These interventions are referred to as "best practices" in patient care. Ongoing analysis enables nurses and other healthcare professionals to "close the gap" between current practice and the "best practices" that are the goals of healthcare provision (Krugman 2003).

A common term used to describe the discrepancies between theory, research, and practice is the "theory-practice" gap. This gap refers to insufficient understanding of the value of theory to clinical practice, a lack of awareness by nurses of the theory that guides nursing practice, and the differences between best practice patient care interventions and the actual patient interventions that are implemented (Billings & Kowalski 2006). Best practices can be implemented only when nurses know what they are and have the resources with which to implement them.

A national database of best practices should be easily accessible to staff nurses, as well as management, administrative, and research personnel. Interpretation of best practices must not be limited to doctorally prepared nurses. All nurses should and must be able to use research findings as part of their practice.

In 1995, the American Nurses Association (ANA) published *Nursing Report Care*, which evolved into the *National Database of Nursing Quality Indicat*ors (Krugman 2003; National Database of Nursing Quality Indicators 2007). This database is an excellent resource for both clinicians and staff development specialists and can be retrieved from *www.nursingquality.org*. Other helpful databases include:

- *The Joanna Briggs Institute, in Adelaide, Australia:* Affiliated with Royal Adelaide Hospital and has a worldwide network of collaborators. The institute provides best-practice information sheets and systematic reviews of nursing topics. *www.joanna briggs.edu.au.*

EVIDENCE-BASED STAFF DEVELOPMENT

- *Worldviews on Evidence-Based Nursing:* Published by Sigma Theta Tau International in both print and electronic format. It presents systematic literature reviews, articles, and abstracts. An online subscription is required to view the articles, which are also available for individual purchase at *www.blackwellpublishing.com/wvn.*

Are such clinical databases useful for the implementation of evidence-based staff development practice? Absolutely. As staff development specialists, we are responsible for offering continuing education that includes information about the latest diagnostic, treatment, preventive, and nursing actions that have a positive impact on patient outcomes.

Since clinical best practice databases are already in existence, it seems logical to incorporate this information into the staff development arena. Let's start by explaining what is meant by the concept of evidence-based staff development practice.

Evidence-based staff development practice

EBP in staff development is the process of using "best practice" evidence to close the gap between actual staff development practice and the identified best practices. But where are these best practices to be found? As noted in Chapter 1, there is a significant lack of staff development research. Without such research, best practices are difficult to identify.

It is, however, possible to use the evidence already available in our various practices. This is not to discount the need for formal research. We can organize the data we have, both to identify best practice methods and to formulate further staff development research studies.

EBP TIP *Needs assessment data and evaluation data can form the foundation of initial EBP in staff development.*

The EBP movement's current emphasis is on clinical practice, and staff development specialists share much of the responsibility for educating nurses and other clinicians regarding its implementation. Knowledge of clinical best practices is essential to program planning.

Fortunately, the National Database of Nursing Quality Indicators (NDNQI) is a good source of nurse-sensitive indicators that reflect the structure, process, and outcome of nursing care (NDNQI 2007).

Information is collected on the following indicators:

- Patient falls
- Pressure ulcers
- Physical/sexual assault
- Pain management
- Peripheral IV infiltration
- Physical restraints
- Staff mix
- Nursing care hours provided per patient day
- RN education/certification
- RN surveys

EBP TIP *For more information about NDNQI, log on to* www.nursingquality.org.

Staff development specialists can use such clinical data to plan educational programs that reflect current best practices. Additionally, they can use evaluation data as evidence to guide program planning. Multiple resources should be assessed when gathering data. The checklist in Figure 2.1 can help you identify and organize sources of data or evidence for planning. The "Data source" column contains the actual source of data; the "Questions to answer" column helps you to analyze the usefulness of your data sources; and the final column, "Comments," allows you to add information specific to your organization or your thoughts on data collection.

Figure 2.1   **Data-gathering for EBP in staff development**

Data source	Questions to answer	Comments
Needs assessments	How are needs assessments conducted? How often are needs assessments conducted? Are learning needs identified by an appropriate number of representatives from all levels of staff? Do learning needs identified by staff reflect learning needs as identified by management, organizational goals, accreditation standards, performance evaluations, and best practices? How are learning needs prioritized?	
Informal conversations	How are informal conversations documented? How are the data from these conversations used as evidence for program planning? How are the data from these conversations validated?	
Performance evaluations	How are staff development products and services revised and/or initiated as a result of performance evaluation data? How are data regarding educational needs relayed to staff development specialists? Is the system for data retrieval consistent and reliable? What is the system for ensuring that employees who need specific education receive it?	
Competency statements	Are competency statements and staff development products and services correlated? Are competency statements correlated with job descriptions? Have staff development competency statements been identified for staff development specialists?	

Figure 2.1 Data-gathering for EBP in staff development (cont.)

Data source	Questions to answer	Comments
Program evaluation data	Are program evaluation data collected that measure reaction, knowledge acquisition, behavior, outcomes, and return on investment (ROI)? According to these data, what impact did staff development products and services have on: • Knowledge acquisition? • Job performance? • Patient outcomes? • ROI?	
Risk management and quality improvement data	How are risk management and quality improvement data used to plan educational offerings? Do staff development specialists serve as risk management and/or quality improvement committee members? How are these data documented in the program planning process?	
Organizational goals and objectives	What is the evidence that staff development products and services correlate with organizational goals and objectives? What data are collected to prove this correlation?	

 EVIDENCE-BASED STAFF DEVELOPMENT

Historical background

It is not enough simply to gather data and attempt to implement staff development EBP. You need to understand the background of the EBP movement and the other concepts that have affected its evolution.

The competency movement

The concept of competency in job performance is not new. In 1978, Dorothy del Bueno stated that the emphasis of nursing practice is to be placed on the desired outcome. Competency assessment is the evaluation of a nurse or other healthcare professional's ability to perform specific tasks or exhibit identified behaviors according to established standards and criteria (Bradely 2003). In other words, evidence is required to prove competency. The clinical competency movement had considerable impact on the delivery of inservice and continuing education.

The ANA's *Nursing: Scope and Standards of Practice* addresses the topic of competence and education in detail. Standards 8 states, "The registered nurse attains knowledge and competency that reflects current nursing practice" (2004). Achievement of this standard is measured by:

- Participation in ongoing educational activities

- Demonstration of a commitment to lifelong learning

- Maintenance of skills and competence by seeking experiences that reflect current practice

- Acquisition of knowledge and skills appropriate to the specialty area of practice

- Maintenance of professional records that provide evidence of competency and lifelong learning

- Maintenance of skills and competence by seeking appropriate formal and independent learning activities

To facilitate achievement of Standard 8, many staff development specialists deliver competency-based education (CBE) to assess and validate competence (Brunt 2007). CBE models gained prominence in the 1960s and have continued to evolve and correlate with research and EBP.

CBE emphasizes outcomes in terms of the learner's ability to safely and accurately perform a task and implement behaviors. Characteristics of CBE include (Brunt 2007):

- Learner-centered philosophy
- Focus on outcomes
- Criterion-reference evaluation
- Real-life orientation
- Flexibility
- Clear standards

Competence also depends on recognizing and implementing best practices in healthcare. Best practices are identified through the research process.

Research

Much of what constitutes best practices has been determined by medical, rather than nursing, research. This is beginning to change, however, and nursing research is evolving into a valued, much-needed specialty.

As long ago as the 1850s, Florence Nightingale compiled data and wrote reports, such as "Notes Affecting the Health, Efficiency, and Hospital Administration of the British Army" (Nightingale, 1992). Over the centuries, Ms. Nightingale's most prominent image was that of the "lady with the lamp," characterized as an angel of mercy. In truth, she was a competent administrator, researcher, and advocate of nursing professionalism.

Doctorally prepared nurses conduct a great deal of the nursing research underway today. However, nurses with varying levels of education can (and do) conduct research, sometimes without even knowing it. For example, how many times have our clinical nursing colleagues proposed a different method of bladder training, positioning, counseling, or assessment based on experience and evaluation of the success of various interventions? The next step is to document these findings so that the evidence of best practices is clear and concise.

Staff development specialists are in a similar position. When an administrator proposes the immediate initiation of a mandatory program in the middle of July via a classroom setting, most

 EVIDENCE-BASED STAFF DEVELOPMENT

staff development specialists instinctively "know" that this will not work. Vacations and other time constraints prohibit attendance in a classroom setting. By waiting a few weeks, the program can be implemented through a more appropriate methodology, and the number of staff members on vacation will decrease. But where is the evidence for these propositions? Just "knowing" by experience is no longer sufficient. We must document our evidence and use it to improve services and justify our decisions.

Evidence-based practice

EBP in nursing evolved from evidence-based medicine, which originated in Canada as a concept for teaching medical students. This movement began in Paris, where some physicians sought truth by systematic patient observation rather than relying on "expert" information. In 1992, Gordon Guyatt of Canada introduced the term "evidence-based medicine" (Pape 2003).

What sources do nurses rely on for their evidence? A recent research study regarding the frequency with which staff nurses used various sources of knowledge identified six top sources. In order of identification, the sources of knowledge are (Brunt 2007):

1. Experience
2. Information learned in nursing school
3. Workplace sources
4. Physician sources
5. Intuition
6. Past usual practice

Experience is the number one knowledge source used by nurses, and it is critical to staff development specialists as well. Although many practitioners may equate experience with intuition, it is more likely based on evidence. Experience involves the observation and implementation of various interventions, and learning which interventions are the most successful. Is this not research? Observing, comparing, and formulating conclusions based on evidence is research. It just needs to be documented, verified, and accepted as reliable evidence with which to guide practice.

Evolution of staff development practice

In the not-so-distant past, staff development specialists were viewed as "older" nurses who had paid their dues as bedside nurses and were now being rewarded with a Monday–Friday job until retirement. Things have clearly changed. Staff development is now a legitimate specialty crucial to the effectiveness of the organization. The following overview of staff development's evolution shows its beginnings and progress to the arena of EBP in staff development (Avillion 2004):

- Staff development originated with Florence Nightingale's efforts to establish training schools for nurses and to improve the delivery of patient care in hospitals. Nightingale encouraged lifelong learning, but formal staff development programs did not exist in the late 1800s and early 1900s.

- The Great Depression of the late 1920s and 1930s forced many nurses to work in hospital settings for the first time since their initial training. Prior to the Depression, most nurses worked in private practice as duty nurses, and nursing students provided the majority of care to inpatients. This influx of nurses into the hospital setting triggered the need for orientation and inservice programs. However, most instruction was provided by the nurse in charge of the nursing units.

- The advent of World War II was the cause of even more dramatic changes. Registered nurses left the hospital setting to serve in the armed forces, and roles for non professional staff evolved. Inactive nurses returned to practice, and a need for refresher courses emerged. The need for continuing education, inservices, on-the-job training, and orientation increased to the point that charge nurses could no longer meet educational needs. It became evident that a new role for nurses specializing in education was evolving.

- The Joint Commission for the Improvement of Care of the Patient proposed in 1953 that a distinct department devoted to the training and continuing education of the nursing department be established. In 1969, the first national conference on continuing education for nurses was sponsored by the Medical College of Virginia, Health Sciences Division of Virginia Commonwealth University.

EVIDENCE-BASED STAFF DEVELOPMENT

• In the 1970s, journals devoted to the specialty of staff development were published, and the Joint Commission on Accreditation of Hospitals mandated that a position to oversee and coordinate staff development activities be established.

• In the 1990s, the ANA published *Roles and Responsibilities for Nursing Continuing Education and Staff Development Across All Settings*, the first *Core Curriculum for Nursing Staff Development* was published, and the American Nurses Credentialing Center offered the first certification examination for nursing continuing education and professional development. Staff development responsibilities expanded to include responsibility for house wide education rather than only for the nursing department; graduate education was usually required for those in charge of staff development services; and the staff development department was expected to justify its existence by demonstrating the impact of education on patient care and organizational effectiveness.

• The 21st-century staff development specialist is expected to be an expert in the process of planning, implementing, and evaluating education. He or she is also expected to provide evidence that education improves patient outcomes in a cost-effective, efficient manner. Hence, the time for EBP in staff development has arrived.

The need for EBP in staff development

The staff development specialty has evolved from an informal process of on-the-job training provided by a charge nurse to a formal system of delivering education that is expected to improve job performance and patient outcomes. Such education is also expected to be provided in a cost-effective manner. All of these expectations require that staff development specialists gather pertinent data and use that data as evidence to justify the way products and services are designed and delivered. The need for evidence increases the necessity for both formal and informal research in the field of staff development.

EBP in staff development and the change process

Evidence-based practice in staff development is a learned skill that requires intellectual curiosity and the desire to explore opportunities. Part of staff development EBP is learning how to question traditional practice and analyze best practice evidence (Penz and Bassendowski 2006).

> **EBP TIP** *Staff development specialists must accept and promote change. Change is a dynamic process that necessitates alterations in behavior, which can cause conflict and/or resistance. Review the change process and determine how your department can best adapt to the changes triggered by the implementation of EBP in staff development.*

Lippitt's seven-step change theory (Dittman 2001; Kritsonis 2004–2005) is particularly appropriate for the implementation of EBP in staff development.

Step 1: Identify change agent(s). Identify problems (or desired new methods of practice) by examining all possible consequences. Determine who will be affected by the changes and who will be responsible for solving the problems or implementing new practice methods. Involve persons to be affected by change in problem resolution and/or implementation of new practice methods. This will ensure that persons affected by the change are committed to its success.

Step 2: Identify the financial and human resources that are needed for the change and determine if they exist within the current organizational structure.

Step 3: Evaluate the change agent(s)'s motivation and resources, experience, stamina, and commitment.

Step 4: Develop action plans and strategies for problem resolution or implementation of new practice methods.

Step 5: Explain the role of the change agent(s) to all affected persons.

Step 6: Establish mechanisms for facilitating feedback, enhancing communication, and coordinating the effects of change.

Step 7: Gradually terminate the helping relationship aspects of the change agent(s).

Figure 2.2 is a template for initiating change. It is based on Lippitt's change theory and is adapted for dealing with changes triggered by the implementation of EBP in staff development. The columns explain options for implementation. Adapt this template to best fit the needs of your department and organization. (Note that the various levels of staff development expertise are discussed in Chapter 1).

2.2   **Dealing with staff development EBP changes**

Steps	Tasks	Responsibility	Special considerations
Step 1: Identify change agent(s) and determine who will be affected by the change	• Select the staff development specialists who will assume primary responsibility for implementing staff development EBP • Compile a list of affected persons/departments with priority given to administration and management since these persons can make or break successful implementation	Manager or director of the staff development department and staff development specialists	The manager is often the primary change agent for this type of major project. If the staff development department is small, all members of the department may have significant responsibility as change agents. Larger departments may have the luxury of assigning primary responsibility for change to proficient or expert staff development specialists, although the entire staff must be involved in the process. If you have staff development specialists of varying levels of expertise, this task may be appropriate for someone at the advanced beginner or competent levels. Novices could work with these individuals to accomplish this task.
Step 2: Identify financial and human resources necessary for change and determine if they currently exist	• Determine current expenses associated with implementation of EBP. Examples of expenses include: - Continuing education in research and EBP - Expenses associated with research projects - Purchase of professional journal subscriptions, books, and other resources pertaining to research, competency, and EBP	Manager or director of the staff development department in conjunction with his or her staff members	It is tempting for the manager to rely on the most experienced staff development specialists for project implementation. It is a serious mistake to overload the most experienced staff members and to overlook those who are less experienced. For change to be successful, *all* members of the department must feel that they are contributing to the success of EBP implementation.

Figure 2.2 **Dealing with staff development EBP changes (cont.)**

Steps	Tasks	Responsibility	Special considerations
	• Identify human resources necessary for successful change (implementation of EBP in staff development) - What are the levels of expertise of the staff development specialists currently employed? What additional training and education are necessary to prepare these persons to successfully implement EBP? - Are members of another department adjunct faculty for staff development? If so, how will they be trained in the delivery of EBP in staff development? - What mechanisms for research are currently in place (e.g., research committees, research departments)? How can you partner with the persons responsible for these endeavors to promote EBP in staff development?		
Step 3: Evaluate the change agent(s)'s motivation, resources, experience, stamina, and commitment	• Determine the level of expertise of each member of the staff development department (see Chapter 1 for assistance) • Determine the level of knowledge concerning staff development EBP • Assess the current workload of each member of the staff development department	Manager or director of the staff development department in conjunction with his or her staff members	The implementation of Step 3 tasks is an excellent opportunity to groom less experienced staff development specialists. They can use opportunities generated by Step 3 tasks to increase their proficiency in staff development practice.

 EVIDENCE-BASED STAFF DEVELOPMENT

2.2   **Dealing with staff development EBP changes (cont.)**

Steps	Tasks	Responsibility	Special considerations
Step 4: Develop action plans and strategies for EBP implementation	• Develop action plan for implementation of EBP in staff development (see Chapter 4 for an action plan template)	All members of the staff development department	If persons from other departments are responsible for implementing certain phases of the action plan, be sure to include them in the development of the plan.
Step 5: Explain the role of the change agent(s) in the implementation of EBP in staff development to all affected persons.	• Develop clear, concise reports to explain and document the advantages of EBP (an example of such a report appears in Chapter 4)	Members of the staff development department who are wellversed and confident in presenting information to administration and management	The manager or director of staff development should assume responsibility for presenting this type of information to administration. Other members of the department who have reached proficient or expert status should work with less experienced staff development specialists.
Step 6: Establish mechanisms for feedback and communicating the effects of change	• Include reports concerning EBP implementation and its effect on the organization in all staff development staff meetings • Include status updates for presentation at department director/management meetings • Incorporate such mechanisms in action plans	All staff development department members	Open communication is essential to the success of staff development EBP. Soon, the organization will become accustomed to hearing staff development reports in an EBP format. Figure 4.1 is a good example of a report written in EBP format.
Step 7: Gradually terminate the helping relationship aspects of the change agent(s)	• Monitor the comfort level of administration, management, and staff with EBP in staff development via communication mechanisms identified in Step 6 • Transition all reports and program planning endeavors into an EBP format	All staff development department members	The staff development is not necessarily terminating a helping relationship. It is helping the organization to recognize the benefits of EBP and become accustomed to thinking and acting in ways that facilitate EBP in both clinical and non-clinical settings.

References

American Nurses Association. (2004). *Nursing: Scope and Standards of Practice.* Washington, DC: ANA.

Avillion, A. E. (2004). *A Practical Guide to Staff Development: Tools and Techniques for Effective Education.* Marblehead, MA: HCPro.

Billings, D., and Kowalski, K. (2006). "Bridging the theory-practice gap with evidence-based practice." *The Journal of Continuing Education in Nursing,* 37(6), 248–249.

Bradely, D. (2003). "Validating competency at the bedside." *Journal for Nurses in Staff Development,* 19(4), 165–175.

Brunt, B. A. (2007). *Competencies for Staff Educators.* Marblehead, MA: HCPro.

del Bueno, D. (1978). "Competency-based education." *Nurse Educator,* 3, 10–14.

Dittman, P. W. (2001). "Change and change agents." A. E. Avillion (Ed.), *Core Curriculum for Staff Development (2nd ed., pp. 97–121).* Pensacola, FL: National Nursing Staff Development Organization.

Kritsonis, A. (2004–2005). "Comparison of change theories." *International Journal of Scholarly Academic Intellectual Diversity,* 8(1).

Krugman, M. (2003). "Evidence-based practice: The role of staff development." *Journal for Nurses in Staff Development,* 19(6), 279–285.

National Database of Nursing Quality Indicators. (2007). Retrieved April 13, 2007 from *www.nursingquality.org.*

EVIDENCE-BASED STAFF DEVELOPMENT

Nightingale, F. (1992). *Notes on Nursing: What It Is and What It Is Not (Commemorative Edition)*. Philadelphia: Lippincott.

Pape, T. M. (2003). "Evidence-based nursing practice: To infinity and beyond." *The Journal of Continuing Education in Nursing, 34(4), 154–161.*

Penz, K. L., & Bassendowski, S. L. (2006). "Evidence-based nursing in clinical practice: implications for nurse educators." *The Journal of Continuing Education in Nursing, 37(6), 250–256.*

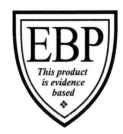

This product
is evidence
based

Implications for
evidence-based staff
development practice

Implications for evidence-based staff development practice

Learning objectives

After reading this chapter, the participant will be able to:

- Discuss the advantages and barriers to evidence-based practice (EBP) in staff development

- Explain the ethical implications of EBP in staff development

- Identify legal implications of EBP in staff development

Before you implement evidence-based staff development practice, it is important that you understand its implications. There are certainly advantages to its implementation, but there are also barriers and ethical and legal issues to consider. The ability to discuss these issues knowledgably will help you to justify EBP in staff development.

Advantages to EBP in staff development

The ultimate advantage of EBP in staff development is the ability to provide high-quality, cost-effective education services that have a knowledge and/or evidence base (Pape 2003). It enables staff development specialists to apply best practices and pertinent research findings to their endeavors.

Another advantage of EBP is bridging the gap between theory and staff development practice (Billings & Kowalski 2006). EBP encourages staff development specialists to participate in and use the findings from research studies. Additional advantages include:

- EBP supports the need for and stimulates interest in the research process. There is a significant lack of formal staff development research. Although informal research is certainly valuable, formal research will not only add to the knowledge base of the specialty, but will increase its credibility in the healthcare community. Implementing EBP requires that staff development specialists augment their knowledge of the research process and their ability to conduct valid and reliable studies.

- It is expected that the implementation of EBP will improve staff development services. It is also expected that improved staff development services will lead to an improvement in the job performance of clinicians and other staff development customers. Ultimately, improved job performance should result in better patient outcomes. Correlation of better patient outcomes to education services is an excellent research project.

- Communication between the staff development department and other departments within the organization is improved through the use of EBP. When justifying educational endeavors, including how and why such endeavors should be offered, the use of evidence can help formulate a persuasive argument. Good communication is the foundation of establishing an EBP culture.

- Implementation of EBP can increase the job satisfaction of all levels of staff development specialists but especially those who have reached the expert level. As in any specialty, there is the danger of becoming bored or "burned out" after performing the same or similar job for a number of years. The implementation of EBP will pose challenges and stimulate new interests among expert practitioners. These practitioners may also assume the role of researcher and add to the body of knowledge regarding staff development practice.

> **EBP TIP** *Credibility in the scientific healthcare community depends, in part, on the identification of a body of knowledge unique to a particular discipline or specialty. Conducting staff development research will help to determine that body of knowledge and garner respect in the healthcare community.*

Barriers to EBP in staff development

It is never easy to implement a new way of conducting business, and you will face barriers to the implementation of EBP in staff development. The first of these is a shortage of staff development research. Many of the research studies conducted by staff development specialists concentrate on clinicians' attitudes toward education or what factors trigger nurses to participate in continuing education, but consider some of these topics:

- What education strategies produce the most efficient application of knowledge in the work setting?

- What education strategies are associated with improved job performance and improved patient outcomes?

- How does education affect the financial status of the organization?

These are just a few ideas that could be refined and expanded upon. You should also consider how you analyze the plethora of data you obtain from needs assessments, program evaluations, and the many other sources identified in Chapter 2. You probably have the foundation for many research explorations, as well as a solid basis for evidence-based practice in staff development.

> **EBP TIP** *Always consider publishing your research findings. It is our responsibility to add to the body of staff development knowledge by sharing our research endeavors. Professional journals such as* The Journal of Continuing Education in Nursing *and* The Journal for Nurses in Staff Development *are devoted to staff development and provide excellent opportunities for publication.*

Brunt's (2007) recently published research findings concerning the identification of valid competencies for staff educators notes that although there is extensive literature devoted to clinical competence, there is only limited literature available on what types of competencies should be achieved by staff development specialists. It is up to us to conduct and analyze the evidence that will guide our staff development practice.

A barrier that is closely linked to the lack of actual staff development research is a lack of knowledge about the research process. Graduate programs generally require students to complete at least one major research project, but this does not qualify them as experts in the research process.

Staff development specialists should pursue continuing education opportunities in the research field. This will help to conduct objective, scientific research studies in the staff development field. Simple research studies, such as the effect of education on patient outcomes, can be organized and conducted with the cooperation of direct patient care providers. Collaboration with your organization's research committee is an excellent way to learn more about research and promote staff development topics as valid research endeavors.

EBP TIP *Consider collaborating with physicians as part of your research endeavors. Identify physicians who have demonstrated interest in both education and research. They would probably be interested in participating in studies that measure the effect of new treatments on patient outcomes. You could combine this with an assessment of how education concerning such treatments impacts these outcomes.*

Another barrier to the implementation of EBP is lack of time. This barrier is twofold: lack of time for accessing, reading, and evaluating research; and lack of time for learning how to conduct, analyze, and apply research findings (Pravikoff, Tanner, & Pierce 2005). No one has the luxury of excessive amounts of time at work or at home. However, it is imperative that time for research-related activities be worked into schedules in the same way time would be made to attend a committee meeting, plan a program, or implement an educational activity. It is the responsibility of the director of the department and her or his staff to learn more about the research process, begin to conduct research, and apply findings to the department's practice.

EBP TIP *Like clinicians, staff development specialists have a responsibility for lifelong learning. One area of continuing education is the research process and how to use research findings to enhance staff development services.*

Staff resistance is another barrier to EBP in staff development. A certain level of resistance may be expected from members of other departments and/or the administration, as they question how EBP will affect their access to education. However, since EBP in the clinical arena is swiftly gaining acceptance, similar changes in staff development practice will also gain acceptance if the rationale for the change is solid and compelling.

A more significant amount of resistance may be displayed by staff development specialists within your own department. Change is difficult and may trigger the following concerns:

- Fear of not being able to comprehend and/or implement EBP in staff development
- Concern that EBP may cause more work
- Fear that EBP may show staff development inadequacies
- Dislike of the research process
- Dislike of theory
- Concern that EBP may lead to a change in roles and responsibilities

These fears, concerns, and dislikes are not unreasonable and require that the person in charge of implementing EBP in staff development (usually the manager or director of the department) provides education about the process and designs a careful plan for its implementation (see Chapter 4). Note that all members of the department will ultimately play a significant part in either its success or its failure.

EBP TIP *Reassure staff development specialists that it is not necessary to hold a doctorate in order to implement EBP effectively in staff development.*

A final barrier to implementation of EBP in staff development is cost. It takes financial resources to conduct research and to allow employees to pursue research, analyze staff development data, and implement changes in practice. However, part of the education process concerning EBP is to show that it will actually increase cost-effectiveness.

EBP TIP *Increase the number of times you determine return on investment (ROI) for particular education programs. This will help to convince doubters of the cost-effectiveness of EBP.*

Ethical implications

Ethical dilemmas can, and do, occur with the implementation of EBP in staff development. For example, suppose that data from coronary care orientation activities show that nurses who fail initial pharmacology and rhythm strip interpretation exams have difficulty assimilating into the critical care arena and terminate employment in less than one year. You have gathered data to support these statements and have calculated the cost of orienting, precepting, and providing additional training for these nurses. You recommend that successful completion of these exams be a prerequisite for continued employment. The coronary care nurse manager, however, resists these requirements. She tells you and the vice president of nursing services that she is short-staffed and that it's better to have employees for a year rather than not at all, despite the costs of orientation, preceptorship, and education.

Ethically, you do not feel that this is a reasonable decision. Not only does it cost the organization a lot of money, it frustrates nurses on the unit who must carry extra workloads while the new nurses attempt to complete orientation; places new nurses in an environment that is likely to result in an unsatisfactory work experience; and wastes the time of preceptors, staff nurses, and staff development specialists. You present your data to the vice president of nursing services. She accuses you of failing to act as a "team player" and mandates that orientation be "less demanding" for nurses new to the coronary care unit.

Sadly, this scenario is not uncommon. Many staff development specialists have been asked to reduce standards or make changes that they know are not in the best interests of the staff member, organization, and/or patients. These kinds of conflicts are referred to as conflicting moral claims, or, in other words, ethical dilemmas. Morals are those personal beliefs of what is right or wrong, or good or bad, in human behavior. Morals are tied to the values, ideals, customs, modes of conduct, and/or goals that are prized and deemed valuable by individuals, groups, or society (Burkhardt & Nathaniel 2002).

Ethics involve the process of making decisions based upon moral beliefs (Burkhardt & Nathaniel 2002). By their very nature, ethical decisions generally have no clear-cut right or wrong answer. In the preceding scenario, the nurse manager and the vice president of nursing services believe that it is best for the unit to hire nurses to lessen staffing shortages, even if data show that it is not cost-efficient or time-efficient for those persons involved in orienting new employees. As the staff development expert, you have gathered evidence that shows the problems with this type of hiring practice. You believe that it is unethical to hire nurses who have a poor chance of success and that it is also unfair to the organization. The manager and vice president believe that it is better to attempt to fill vacancies under any circumstances. Who is right? Who is wrong?

In most cases, objective evidence helps all involved persons to come to a consensus. However, in some cases, ethical dilemmas persist. It can be quite frustrating to the staff development specialist who has taken the time to implement an evidence-based practice to find that opposition exists despite such evidence. The staff development department must be willing to contend with ethical dilemmas and continue to promote what is best for the organization, its employees, and the patients.

Legal implications

Most staff development specialists are familiar with the legal implications of clinical practice. They know that they must function within the guidelines of their education, training, licensure, and nurse practice acts. They know that they must adhere to their organizations' policies and procedures, but they must also function within the legal limits of staff development practice as supported by knowledge and evidence.

Staff development specialists must also be familiar with licensure and practice acts of the healthcare professionals and workers that they educate. Licensure and practice act guidelines vary from state to state. It may be perfectly legal to teach certified nursing assistants to administer some types of medications in some states, but it may be illegal in others. The same thing applies to various types of assessment and procedures. You are legally accountable for what you teach; this includes recognizing the mandates of various licensing bodies and practice acts. Let's review a few legal concepts and apply them to EBP in staff development (Follin 2004).

- **Malpractice:** Wrongful conduct, failure to properly discharge professional duties, or failure to meet standards of care that result in harm to another person

- **Liability:** Legal responsibility for the failure to act or taking action that does not meet standards of care, thus causing harm to another person

- **Negligence:** Failure to exercise the degree of care that a "reasonable person of ordinary prudence would exercise under the same circumstances"

In a court of law, four elements must be shown before a healthcare professional is said to be liable for malpractice. These are (Follin 2004):

- **Duty:** There must be a duty owed to the person harmed and the extent of that duty must be shown

- **Breach of duty:** The professional must have failed to competently fulfill his or her duty

- **Causation:** What the professional did or failed to do must be directly linked to the harm that occurred

- **Harm:** It must be shown that injury or harm resulted from the healthcare professional's actions or from failure to act appropriately

Now what does this have to do with evidence-based practice? Consider this scenario. Evidence shows that a specific education program does not have the desired effect on a nurse's behavior in the work setting. Program attendees do not implement new behaviors in the work setting, and failure to implement these behaviors is linked to an increase in nosocomial infections. Analysis indicates that specific changes in methodology and content must be made. However, due to lack of time and other priorities, these changes are not made. A patient develops a serious nosocomial infection and dies. The nurses providing direct care to that patient are found to be negligent, and so is the staff development specialist responsible for planning, implementing, and evaluating that particular program. Evidence showed that a reasonable, prudent staff development specialist would have analyzed data and used the resulting evidence to make necessary program changes.

Evidence-based practice has not only the potential to improve practice and patient outcomes, but also the responsibility to adhere to a high standard of program delivery. Staff development specialists are not exempt from legal responsibility for their products and services.

In summary, there are huge implications for the implementation of evidence-based practice in staff development. Figure 3.1 offers a template for assessing which implications carry the most impact for you and your department and a format for dealing with them.

| Figure 3.1 | Assessing evidence-based implications | |

Implications	Questions for analysis	Comments
Advantages	Is staff development research currently being conducted? If so, what projects are underway? How is staff development data being collected? What is the level of knowledge about the research process among staff development specialists? What is the current status of communication between the staff development department and other departments within the organization?	
Barriers	Who among the staff development specialists shows a particular interest in or aptitude for implementing evidence-based practice in staff development? Who among the staff development specialists is able to interpret research findings accurately? What continuing education programs concerning EBP and research are available? What support exists among managers throughout the organization and administration for the implementation of EBP in staff development? Is there any resistance to implementing EBP among the staff development specialists? If so, what are the reasons for the resistance? What are the estimated costs associated with implementation of EBP in staff development?	
Ethical implications	Do staff development specialists understand the ethical implications for EBP in staff development? What opportunities exist for the staff development specialists to discuss potential or actual ethical dilemmas and possible solutions to these dilemmas? Are there continuing education opportunities in the field of ethics for staff development specialists?	

3.1   **Assessing evidence-based implications (cont.)**

Implications	Questions for analysis	Comments
Legal implications	Are staff development specialists familiar with basic legal terminology? Do they comprehend the four elements of negligence? Do they comprehend their legal obligations concerning staff development products and services? What opportunities are available for staff development specialists to discuss potential legal ramifications of EBP in staff development? What continuing education opportunities are available for staff development specialists regarding legal implications of EBP?	

EVIDENCE-BASED STAFF DEVELOPMENT

References

Billings, D., & Kowalski, K. (2006). "Bridging the theory-practice gap with evidence-based practice." *The Journal of Continuing Education in Nursing*, 37(6), 248–249.

Brunt, B. (2007). *Competencies for Staff Educators: Tools to Evaluate and Enhance Nursing Professional Development*. Marblehead, MA: HCPro.

Burkhardt, M. A., & Nathaniel, A. K. (2002). *Ethics & Issues in Contemporary Nursing* (2nd ed.). Clifton Park, NY: Delmar.

Follin, S. A. (Ed.) (2004). *Nurse's Legal Handbook* (5th ed.). Philadelphia: Lippincott Williams & Wilkins.

Pape, T. M. (2003). "Evidence-based nursing practice: To infinity and beyond." *The Journal of Continuing Education in Nursing*, 34(4), 154–161.

Pravikoff, D. S., Tanner, A. B., & Pierce, S. T. (2005). "Readiness of U.S. nurses for evidence-based practice." *The American Journal of Nursing*, 105(9), 40–52.

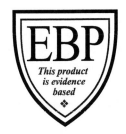

Implementation of
evidence-based practice
in staff development

Implementation of evidence-based practice in staff development

Learning objectives

After reading this chapter, the participant will be able to:

- Explain how to acquire support from staff, management, and administration for the implementation of evidence-based practice (EBP) in staff development

- Formulate strategies for the implementation of EBP in staff development

- Explain how EBP in staff development helps to achieve and maintain Magnet® status

Getting the "buy in" for EBP in staff development

You may know that EBP is the most efficient and cost-effective way to deliver staff development products and services. But how do you convince other members of the staff development department? How do you convince colleagues from other departments, including management and administration? Let's approach this challenge from the perspective of the director of the staff development department.

First, look at your organizational and departmental structure. A one-person staff development department means that one individual is both manager and staff. In a larger department, multiple people are involved in delivering staff development products and services. It is important that those outside the department support EBP, but it is even more important that all members of the staff development department do so. As noted in Chapter 3, one of the most significant barriers to implementation is resistance by staff development specialists themselves.

"Buy in" from staff development specialists

As the leader in the EBP movement, prepare carefully for a meeting with your staff. All staff development specialists are likely familiar with EBP in the clinical setting, so this will not be a totally foreign concept. However, implementing *staff development* EBP is another matter. The fears discussed in the previous chapter are very real and may trigger considerable resistance. Here are some suggestions for preparing your staff to implement EBP:

- **Provide a comfortable environment:** Present the information in a relaxed atmosphere where staff members feel free to ask questions and make comments. Don't squeeze the concept in at the end of a regular staff meeting. Make this presentation a separate, positive event. Include handouts or other audiovisuals, and offer refreshments. This is a change to be celebrated.

- **Ensure consistency of definition:** Make sure everyone is defining EBP in staff development the same way.

- **Ensure consistency of goals:** Work with your staff to formulate realistic goals. Never establish goals in isolation.

- **Identify advantages:** Be sure to explain the advantages of implementing EBP. Include the advantages to the department, to the organization, and to the individual staff development specialists.

- **Identify barriers:** It is as important to identify barriers as it is to identify advantages. Your staff will react negatively if they believe that you are attempting to avoid discussing the problems associated with implementation.

- **Answer questions honestly:** Encourage questions and facilitate discussion. Be supportive, but do not allow members of the department to sabotage the implementation of EBP. Implementation is essential to the growth (and even the survival) of the staff development department. Some resistance to change is normal, and some degree of fear (e.g., fear of change, fear of inability to acquire new skills, fear of changes in responsibilities) is also normal. Sabotage is not.

EBP TIP *Use the templates in Chapters 2 and 3 to identify data resources and the implications of EBP. This will help you to identify many facets of the EBP concept in a logical manner. You can bring completed templates to your staff meeting. This will help you to share your ideas and stimulate discussion.*

Depending on the knowledge base of your staff, you may be able to start developing your action plan at the preliminary meeting. You will need to gauge the comfort level of your staff. They may or may not be ready to commit themselves to a written action plan at this point. It might be wiser to assign specific, limited tasks to be completed prior to the next EBP implementation meeting. Such tasks might include:

- Review the staff development literature for relevant research findings, and present the findings from a relevant study at the next meeting.

- Review data collection methods for a specific area of responsibility (e.g., orientation, mandatory training, a particular continuing education program) and analyze their effectiveness. Present findings at the next implementation meeting.

- Identify research topics relevant to the department and propose initiation of an appropriate research project.

- Seek out continuing education opportunities for staff development specialists pertaining to EBP, research, and evaluation of staff development products and services.

"Buy in" from other departments and administration

It is doubtful that other departments will have terribly strong feelings about EBP in your department. Clinical EBP has undoubtedly been implemented to some extent in your organization, so the concept is not new. The managers and staff of the departments for which you provide staff development services will probably want to know:

- Will my staff members still receive the education and training that they need?

- Will this training and education be effective and convenient?

- Will EBP in staff development facilitate achieving and maintaining necessary accreditations?

- Will the staff development department require more financial resources to implement EBP? (This is a normal question since every department wants more, not less, money to operate. They want to be sure that your department will not take financial resources away from them.)

You will be able to assure your colleagues that EBP will enhance communication and services. In fact, you may be able to collaborate on some research studies that will benefit all departments involved.

Administration will share the same concerns as other departments, but with an emphasis on the financial aspects. Administration will concentrate on the ultimate achievements of EBP: improved services and communication, increased cost-effectiveness, and facilitation of achieving and maintaining various accreditations. Use the preceding questions to guide you in preparing an explanation and justification of the conversion to EBP in staff development.

You may want to relay information to administration using a template that identifies how evidence is used in your program planning, implementation, and evaluation. Figure 4.1 is an example of such a template.

Evidence-Based Staff Development

Figure 4.1   **Administrative report on staff development EBP**

Program title	Needs assessment data	Implementation method(s) and rationale	Evaluation data
Pathophysiology of spinal cord injury (SCI): How to intervene for maximum patient outcomes	80% of RNs working on SCI unit requested update on this topic on annual needs assessment survey. Nurse managers of the neuro-rehabilitation units noted that they documented a need for increased knowledge and application of knowledge concerning pathophysiology of SCI on 55% of RN performance evaluations. Length of stay for SCI patients on these units was four to seven days longer than estimated in 60% of patients. Special comments: The SCI rehabilitation program is relatively new; it has existed for 18 months. 50% of the RNs are new to this specialty.	The program consists of blended learning: a computer-based learning (CBL) component and skills demonstration component. Rationale: The decision for blended learning was based on a pilot study of two groups of RNs: Group I's continuing education was presented entirely in the classroom setting. Group II participated in CBL for the didactic portion of the course and then attended a skills lab. Successful completion of posttests and skills demonstration were as follows: Group I: 90% Group II: 95% Minor adjustments were made to the program, including better opportunities for question-and-answer sessions.	This program was offered over a period of six months. Ninety percent of RNs working on the neuro-rehabilitation units attended this program. One hundred percent of participants successfully completed the post test and skills demonstration lab. Direct observation of nurses who attended the program found that 90% applied new knowledge and skills in the work setting. Length of stay for SCI patients were as estimated upon admission to the SCI program for 98% of patients admitted following implementation of this education program. Two percent of patients had longer than estimated lengths of stay compared to 60% prior to program implementation.

Using this type of format allows you to quickly show not only how and why you made programming decisions based on available evidence but the positive impact education had on a specific patient outcome. There is no guesswork. All comments are backed up by evidence.

The implementation process

"What is the difference between EBP and simply using data from program evaluations to plan and revise staff development products and services?"

This is a reasonable question. The evaluation process is essential to EBP. However, it is the way we use evaluation data, as well as the emphasis on research, that differentiates traditional staff development from EBP. As you analyze your current practice and form an EBP implementation plan, the distinction between the two will become clearer.

Analysis of current practice

The foundation of EBP is the evidence that guides your practice. You need to look at your current method of service delivery and determine how much of it is evidence based, where the evidence comes from, and how that evidence is used. Conduct your analysis formally via a written action plan.

Start by identifying major staff development products and services, such as orientation, mandatory training, and major, ongoing continuing education programs. You cannot simultaneously analyze every product and service that you provide. Start with those programs that have the greatest impact on organizational functioning. These are probably the programs that have the biggest impact on job performance and patient outcomes.

Divide responsibility for analysis among the staff development specialists. Logically, the person or persons who have primary responsibility for particular programs should analyze these services. Figure 4.2 serves as a template for analysis. The template consists of three columns: "Tasks, Findings, and Comments/recommended revisions".

Let's review the template and determine how to use it for analysis. The first section involves data identification. Initial identification should have been accomplished using Figure 2.1, but that is a general form that guides you in identifying all sources of data for staff development products and services. Figure 4.2 is a template for individual program analysis.

EVIDENCE-BASED STAFF DEVELOPMENT

Figure 4.2   **Program analysis template**

Task	Findings	Comments/recommended revisions
Identify: • Existing data sources • Method of collecting data • Method of documenting data • Frequency of data collection • Additional sources of data that need to be, but are not currently, in use		
Describe: • The mechanism for analyzing data and how often this occurs • Frequency of program revisions based on identified evidence		
Determine: • Best practices identified via data analysis • Benchmarks compiled from best practices		
Verify conclusions by: • Reviewing history of best practice conclusions • Reviewing the literature to verify conclusions • Identifying current or potential research projects that correlate with best practices and benchmarks		

Identification of data sources

Specific tasks are listed in the task column. These include identification of existing sources (for the particular program being analyzed), the procedure or method of data collection, how the procedure or method is documented, and how often data is collected. These tasks all deal with the present. They will enable the person responsible for the analysis to evaluate the existing procedures of data collection and analyze their effectiveness. The "Findings" column allows you to record your conclusions in close conjunction with tasks performed. The final column allows you to make additional comments and—of paramount importance—any revisions you would like to make to existing methods and procedures. The last task in this section is to identify additional sources of data that are not currently utilized. This will help you to identify necessary revisions and/or additions.

Description of current data analysis

The previous section concentrates on the mechanics of data collection. This section asks you to describe the mechanism used to analyze data and how often such analysis occurs. This enables you to determine the effectiveness of the procedure you are currently using and think about ways to improve it.

Determination of best practices and benchmarks

The next section of the template requires that you identify best practices in program development and implementation. These best practices may involve teaching/learning methodologies associated with improved job performance or the identification of presenter characteristics associated with high rates of learner application of new knowledge and skills in the work setting.

Best practices cannot be selected from a one-time data analysis. One of the purposes of this template is to identify patterns from data analysis. You will be able to determine what works and what does not regarding the provision of staff development products and services. It is much easier to do this when relying on objective data analysis that produces evidence to support your decisions.

EBP TIP *One of the advantages of using a template is that all members of the staff development department have an opportunity to gather evidence for the identification of best practices.*

Benchmarks are achievements or accomplishments that serve as standards of practice for others to emulate. The benchmarks you identify may serve as standards of practice for staff development specialists from other organizations. Before you can identify benchmarks, you need to be sure that your successes and accomplishments are consistent achievements. For example, suppose you have revised the teaching methodology for a particular program. The first time staff members attend the revised program, knowledge acquisition increases, as well as application of that knowledge in the work setting. You are pleased, but cannot identify the revisions as either best practices or benchmarks. These improvements need to be consistent over a period of time, which is determined on an individual basis depending on how often the program is presented and how consistent the outcomes prove to be.

EBP TIP *A history of best practices helps to validate the selection of benchmarks. They must stand the test of time and multiple participants.*

Verification of conclusions

Next, you are asked to verify or support your conclusions by reviewing a history of best practices. This can be accomplished in a variety of ways, such as reviewing staff development literature and discussing your findings with colleagues both within and outside of your organization.

EBP TIP *Consider publishing your best practice findings or benchmark identification in one of the staff development journals, such as* The Journal of Continuing Education in Nursing *or* The Journal for Nurses in Staff Development.

Identification of research projects

Use this template to identify research projects that correlate with best practices and benchmarks. You may wish to compare the effectiveness of a classroom setting versus distance learning. You will assess not only participant satisfaction but application of knowledge, job performance, and/or patient outcomes. Findings may show that participants dislike distance learning, but that both methods are equally effective and one takes less time and money to produce and implement. This is simple but valuable research, and it will help to justify a particular methodology. Take the time as a department to identify what to study and how best to accomplish the investigation.

Restructure the way staff development conducts business

Figure 4.2 serves as a template for both initial and ongoing program analysis. The staff development department should hold regular staff meetings during which the word "evidence" is prominent.

Staff development specialists should come to each meeting prepared to discuss strengths and weaknesses of their program implementation. These discussions must be supported by evidence. Evidence must also be used to develop new programs. Consider this scenario:

You are asked to implement a program that helps healthcare professionals effectively defuse verbal agitation, after risk management and quality improvement data indicates an increase in adverse occurrences involving verbally abusive patients and visitors. Administration wants the program to be delivered via a written self-learning module. You believe that this type of program is more effective when delivered in a classroom setting with opportunities for discussion and role-play. How do you justify your beliefs?

Use your template to gather data. Have you already conducted programs that require such role-play and discussion? Analyze data and determine best practice evidence. But what if this is a new type of program? In this case, you can conduct a literature review and a review of best practices or benchmarks from other organizations. If you anticipate similar program needs on an ongoing basis, conduct a mini–research investigation. Implement the program via the classroom setting and develop a self-learning module containing the same information with opportunities to select appropriate interactions. Compare the effectiveness of knowledge acquisition, knowledge application, and patient outcomes. In this way, you are finding evidence to support (or not support) your initial reactions.

Writing an action plan

Though it is impossible to develop a template that meets the needs of all staff development departments, it is possible to provide a template that serves as a general guideline when writing your own action plan for the implementation of EBP in staff development.

Figure 4.3 is a proposed action plan template, consisting of five columns titled "Objective," "Actions," "Responsibility," "Target date," and "Evaluation:"

- The "Objective" column identifies specific, measurable outcomes to be achieved.

- The "Actions" column lists the exact tasks that must be performed to achieve each objective.

© 2007 HCPro, Inc. **EVIDENCE-BASED STAFF DEVELOPMENT**

- The "Responsibility" column identifies who is responsible for performing the actions that lead to achievement of the objectives.

- The "Target date" column identifies the desired date of objective achievement.

- The "Evaluation" column is used to document analysis of the success (or lack of success) in achieving objectives. The action plan is revised, as necessary, based on the evaluation of objective achievement.

EBP TIP *The objectives are identified in order of priority. However, you may wish to revise these priorities based on your own departmental and organizational needs. Figure 4.3 contains some suggestions for writing your action plan in the evaluation column. These are not to be taken as actual evaluation statements, but ideas regarding objective achievement.*

4.3   **Action plan**

Objective	Actions	Responsibility	Target date	Evaluation
Identify the person responsible for successful implementation of EBP in staff development				The person who is ultimately responsible is the manager or director of the staff development department.
Educate staff development specialists to implement EBP in staff development				Specific actions and target dates will depend on the size of the department and the expertise of its staff. Earlier in this chapter there are specific suggestions for helping your staff to embrace the concept of EBP in staff development.
Evaluate the staff development specialists' motivation for, experience with, and commitment to EBP in staff development				This is the responsibility of the manager or director of the staff development department.
Identify those persons outside the staff development department who will be affected by the implementation of EBP in staff development				This is a fairly easy task and should be quickly accomplished. Remember that Figure 2.2 is a useful resource when writing your action plan.
Determine the implications of implementing EBP in staff development				Figure 3.1 will help you to accomplish this objective. It also offers suggestions for overcoming barriers and resistance to the implementation of EBP in staff development. If significant barriers are identified, you may want to write an objective specific to overcoming these barriers.

 EVIDENCE-BASED STAFF DEVELOPMENT

Figure 4.3   **Action plan (cont.)**

Objective	Actions	Responsibility	Target date	Evaluation
Identify data resources for the implementation of EBP in staff development				Use Figure 2.1 to accomplish this objective. Note that less experienced staff development specialists might benefit from assuming this responsibility with guidance from their more experienced colleagues.
Explain the rationale for implementing EBP in staff development to administration, management, and staff members				Suggestions for achieving this objective appear earlier in this chapter. It is highly recommended that you present data in an objective form, such as that in Figure 4.1. This format can be adapted to present information to various groups.
Analyze current staff development products and services for the transition to staff development EBP				Analysis should help you to identify best practices and possible research topics. Figure 4.2 is a template for analysis that will help you to achieve this objective.
Revise staff development products and services based on evidence				This objective will be ongoing since the staff development specialty should constantly undergo improvement. Analysis and revisions should become part of staff development quality indicators.
Establish a mechanism for identification of best practices and research topics				This should include collaboration with staff development specialists from other organizations. Working together and sharing knowledge will prove to be beneficial to everyone.

4.3 Action plan (cont.)

Objective	Actions	Responsibility	Target date	Evaluation
Complete a staff development research investigation for the purpose of identifying a best practice for a critical product or service				Achievement of this objective will depend on staff expertise and collaboration with other staff development specialists.
Revise or write policies and procedures to reflect EBP in staff development				Responsibility for this objective should be distributed.
Revise staff development staff meeting format so that reports, suggestions, proposals, etc., are based on evidence				Use and revise the templates in this book to help you establish your own user-friendly format.
Communicate the results of EBP in staff development to administration, management, and colleagues				This communication should allow for the expression of questions and concerns. It should also be used to demonstrate how staff development products and services impact job performance and patient outcomes. Nothing sells a new idea like evidence of positive impact.

EVIDENCE-BASED STAFF DEVELOPMENT

ANCC Magnet Recognition Program® status and EBP in staff development

The desired outcomes of ANCC Magnet Recognition Program® status and EBP in staff development are remarkably similar. The achievement of Magnet designation and the implementation of EBP should lead to an improvement in practice environments, job performance, quality of care, and patient outcomes. In fact, the two are interrelated, and EBP can facilitate the journey toward Magnet status.

The Magnet Recognition Program stresses the importance of research to clinical practice. Descriptive research conducted by Magnet Recognition Status organizations produce "a body of knowledge that define the practice environments with them" (Turkel 2004). Staff development should add to that body of knowledge.

There are 14 Forces of Magnetism derived from research conducted in the original Magnet-status hospitals. These Forces are the characteristics that differentiate Magnet-designated hospitals from non-Magnet-designated hospitals and enabled the originally designated hospitals to recruit and retain nurses (Turkel 2004). Let's review these Forces and how EBP can facilitate their integration into nursing practice.

Force of Magnetism 1: Quality of nursing leadership

In Magnet-designated hospitals, nurse leaders are advocates for, and supportive of, their nursing staff. Examples of appropriate nurse leader behaviors that are facilitated by EBP in staff development include:

- **Establishing a shared governance and collaborative practice environment that is in place, and not merely a theoretical concept.** EBP enables staff development specialists to collaborate with the nursing department to implement shared governance. Such collaboration is enhanced by education that is effective and outcome oriented. EBP helps to identify best practices in education that, in turn, will facilitate an appropriate practice environment.

- **Assisting all levels of nursing staff to publish.** EBP enables staff development specialists to conduct research, identify best practices, determine benchmarks, and publish these results in professional journals. Staff development specialists will also develop educational programs to help nurses write articles for publication.

- **Facilitating nursing research and the implementation of clinical EBP.** Staff development specialists are often instrumental to the successful establishment of clinical EBP. Demonstration of EBP in staff development—and how such practice enhances job performance—contributes to a successful nursing environment (Turkel 2004).

Force of Magnetism 2: Organizational structure

Organizational structures are generally flat, with an emphasis on unit decision-making. Executive leaders of the nursing department serve at the executive level of the organization. It is important that staff nurses are involved in organizational meetings and interdisciplinary committees. Shared governance is in place and unit-based advisory councils exist. Staff nurses must also be involved in quality improvement, leadership, recruitment and retention, and educational endeavors (Turkel 2004).

Staff development EBP provides a knowledge and evidence-based foundation for education planning and implementation that demonstrates staff nurses' (and other clinicians') involvement in the education process. Since communication is an integral part of achieving and maintaining Magnet status, the improved communication that accompanies EBP is sure to enhance an organization's pursuit of Magnet designation.

EBP TIP *When gathering data and documenting evidence, consider assessing the effectiveness of staff nurses as partners in the education process, whether it be as planners, teachers, and/or evaluators.*

Force of Magnetism 3: Management style

Organizations rely on a participative management style rather than a manager-focused style. Feedback from all levels of staff is encouraged and valued. The chief nursing executive is available round-the-clock at various times to listen to staff nurses' ideas and concerns. Unit-based governance councils are in place and functioning, peer evaluations are conducted, and staff meeting minutes reflect staff nurse input and feedback (Turkel 2004).

EBP in staff development requires that evidence of communication regarding effectiveness of education be documented. This includes data analysis, determination of evidence, and program revision based on evidence. All of these processes include documentation of staff nurses' (and other clinicians') participation and documentation of how education influenced their job performance and patient outcomes.

Force of Magnetism 4: Personnel policies and programs

Characteristics of policies and programs include (Turkel 2004):

- Competitive salaries and benefits

- Flexible staff models

- Staff involvement in the creation of personnel policies

- Evidence of opportunities for growth and advancement in administration and clinical areas

Projects include new nurse graduate internships, opportunities for continuing education, and student nurse extern programs. The staff development department is intricately involved in all three of these areas. Surveyors expect that intern and extern programs are assessed, and evidence exists that supports the way programs are planned, implemented, and evaluated. Surveyors also expect to see an organized system for the needs assessment, planning, implementation, and evaluation of educational endeavors. The fact that the department focuses on knowledge- and/or research-based evidence is a plus.

Force of Magnetism 5: Professional models of care

Models of care give nurses responsibility and authority for the provision of direct patient care (Turkel 2004). Primary care models and evidence of interdisciplinary collaboration are important. EBP in staff development allows for a continuous circle of feedback among departments and between nurses. Evidence is available to explain how decisions are made regarding staff development products and services, as well as how all levels of staff contribute to educational design. Again, evidence helps to prove that the organization encourages communication and bases its behaviors on this evidence.

Force of Magnetism 6: Quality of care

High-quality patient care is the organizational priority. We have discussed the importance of ensuring that education offerings have a positive impact on job performance and patient outcomes. A system that can provide evidence that education has a positive impact on knowledge acquisition, knowledge application in the work setting, and improved patient outcomes as a result of such application is a huge advantage when applying for Magnet status.

Force of Magnetism 7: Quality improvement

Organizations view quality improvement as educational, and staff nurse participation in the quality process is essential (Turkel 2004). EBP requires that staff development specialists function as members of the quality improvement team; gather data from quality findings; and use that data as evidence when planning, implementing, and evaluating programs. Again, EBP documentation helps to illustrate the circle of communication among departments, particularly nursing. Educational needs regarding quality improvement are communicated and documented as a result of nursing and staff development involvement in the process.

Force of Magnetism 8: Consultation and resources

Facilities provide adequate consultation and human resources, including advanced practice nurses. Peer support is essential (Turkel 2004). Project examples include:

- Availability of advanced practice nurses for consultation
- Staff nurse representation on the ethics committee
- Adequate literature resources (e.g., journals, hospital library, computer programs)
- Flexible and easily accessible education

Staff development specialists can act as consultants to staff nurses who want to publish and who are interested in collaborating on research projects. The effectiveness of a variety of methods of education (e.g., distance learning, classroom learning, nursing rounds) is assessed and documented and used as evidence of compliance.

EBP TIP *Involve staff nurses in research efforts when you are assessing the impact of educational programs on patient outcomes and job performance.*

Force of Magnetism 9: Autonomy

Nurses are expected to practice autonomously and exercise independent judgment within the guidelines of professional standards and licensure. Helping nurses to progress in knowledge and comfort with decision-making coincides with education. Nurses need help to move from the novice to the expert area. We need to plan education programs that help them to do this, and the success of such efforts must be assessed and evidence gathered to prove the impact of these programs.

Force of Magnetism 10: Community and the hospital

Outreach programs exist that result in the organization being perceived as a strong, positive presence in the community. Such programs often include patient education efforts. Staff

EVIDENCE-BASED STAFF DEVELOPMENT

development specialists may also function as patient educators and/or help staff nurses to learn the art of the teaching/learning process so that they become more effective patient educators. Remember that the effectiveness of patient education must be assessed, just as the effectiveness of continuing education is assessed within the organization. Patient outcomes serve as evidence of program effectiveness. Additionally, staff development specialists should seek out opportunities to work as part of the community presence instead of waiting to be asked.

EBP TIP *Outreach programs serve as excellent opportunities for collaborative research between staff nurses and staff development specialists. Think about comparing various patient education methods to determine which is most effective and results in the best patient outcomes.*

Force of Magnetism 11: Nurses as teachers

Nurses are expected to incorporate teaching in all aspects of their practice (Turkel 2004). Examples of the teacher role include:

- Preceptor
- Patient educator
- Mentor
- Teacher of colleagues and subordinates

Most staff nurses do not have a background or training in the teaching/learning process, and so staff development specialists have an important role to play in developing these new educators. They may function as patient educators but are also expected to educate staff nurses in the teaching/learning process. This education should be assessed for effectiveness. In other words, what is the evidence that the staff nurses are effective patient educators as a result of being trained in the teaching/learning process?

Force of Magnetism 12: Image of nursing

Nurses are viewed as essential to the organization by administration and other members of the healthcare team (Turkel 2004). Staff development specialists may help to enhance the image of nursing by facilitating research, publication, and nurse involvement in organizational committees and presentations at national conferences and conventions.

Force of Magnetism 13: Interdisciplinary relationships

Mutual respect among all disciplines exists throughout the organization. From the staff development perspective, mutual respect is demonstrated during the planning, implementation, and evaluation of education endeavors. Cooperation, collaborative research, and data collection should involve members of the interdisciplinary team. Evidence of this should be documented following the analysis of education programs.

Force of Magnetism 14: Professional development

Staff development responsibilities are most prominent in this Force. It is required that opportunities exist for competency-based clinical advancement; that resources are available to maintain competency; and that flexible, relevant, effective continuing education and inservice programs are offered. A particularly strong emphasis is placed on orientation, inservices, continuing education, formal education, and career development.

EBP in staff development will allow surveyors to not only observe a system of education, but examine evidence pertaining to the effectiveness of education offerings. They will also be able to see how evidence is used to improve services.

EBP TIP *When preparing for Magnet status designation, incorporate evidence-based terminology in your discussions with colleagues. This will allow you to become comfortable with justifying your efforts in objective terms.*

Reference

Turkel, M. C. (2004). *Magnet Status: Assessing, Pursuing, and Achieving Nursing Excellence.* Marblehead, MA: HCPro.

EVIDENCE-BASED STAFF DEVELOPMENT

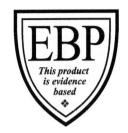

Using evaluation data as part of evidence-based practice in staff development

Using evaluation data as part of evidence-based practice in staff development

Learning objectives

After reading this chapter, the participant will be able to:

- Apply program evaluation data to evidence-based practice (EBP) in staff development

Review of evaluation procedure

It wasn't so long ago that program evaluations consisted primarily of reactive types of data: Was the instructor interesting? Was the instructor knowledgeable? Was the classroom comfortable?

Then, as healthcare became as much a business as a service industry, everything changed. Education was viewed as a luxury, not a necessity, and downsizing hit the staff development department particularly hard. Fortunately for us, staff development specialists learned to expand their evaluation process to include measurement of knowledge acquisition, knowledge application in the job setting, impact of education on patient and organizational outcomes, and return on investment (ROI).

Gathering these types of evaluation data is still necessary. It is how we use them that has changed. We need to think in terms of evidence, not just data. Gathering and analyzing these data can be the foundation of a variety of research projects. The purpose here is to explain how to apply program evaluation data to EBP in staff development.

Analyzing reactive data

Figure 5.1 offers a template for obtaining reactive data, or the learner's reaction to and satisfaction with a learning activity offered in a classroom setting. Figure 5.2 is a template for obtaining reactive data from a distance learning activity. Both are reprinted from the *Nurse Educator Manual*, published by HCPro, Inc.

Consider this scenario:

Amy is the staff development specialist responsible for continuing education offerings for nurses who work on a women's oncology unit. Of particular interest and importance are a series of programs dealing with treatment advances in breast cancer. One of the programs focuses on chemotherapy and is presented by a well-known oncologist, Mark Bowman, MD. Participants complain that his teaching style is boring and that they hate having to sit through his classes. They do note, however, that his handouts are excellent and he makes time for extensive question-and-answer periods. Due to scheduling difficulties, another oncologist, Teresa Mason, MD, is assigned to teach some of the classes. Dr. Mason relies on Dr. Bowman's handouts as a guide for instruction. Her teaching style is lively and entertaining, and participants react favorably to her as a presenter. Amy is considering asking Dr. Mason to teach all of the classes. As Amy puts it, "The data show that Dr. Mason is a better teacher." Is this evidence? Is this a good decision? What would you do?

EBP mandates that you analyze your data to produce objective evidence for your decisions. Available reactive data show that Dr. Mason is the more popular presenter, but this does not mean that education is more effective when she is the instructor. Reactive data alone does not justify major program changes. Amy needs to look at data that measure knowledge acquisition, knowledge application, and, if available, impact on patient outcomes. After collecting these data, Amy can produce evidence to justify any program changes.

As it turns out, knowledge acquisition measured via a pre- and post test is the same regardless of whether Dr. Bowman or Dr. Mason teaches the class. However, nurses who attended Dr. Bowman's classes applied their new knowledge in the work setting more consistently than those

Figure 5.1   Classroom evaluation form

Date: _____

Time: _____

Name (optional): _____

Profession: _____

Department/unit: _____

Program title: _____

Instructor(s): _____

Objectives:

     1.
     2.
     3.

Please answer the following questions: (Note: N/A stands for not applicable)

1. How well did the program content meet the stated objectives?
    __Excellent __Very good __Good __Fair __Poor __N/A

2. Based on the program content, how well were you able to achieve the objectives?
    a. Objective #1_____
        __Excellent __Very good __Good __Fair __Poor __N/A

    b. Objective #2_____
        __Excellent __Very good __Good __Fair __Poor __N/A

    c. Objective #3_____
        __Excellent __Very good __Good __Fair __Poor __N/A

3. Was the instructor an effective teacher?
    __Excellent __Very good __Good __Fair __Poor __N/A

4. Was the instructor knowledgeable and well prepared to teach this program?
    __Excellent __Very good __Good __Fair __Poor __N/A

5. Was there enough time for discussion and to ask questions?
    __Excellent __Very good __Good __Fair __Poor __N/A

5.1　　　　　　　　　　**Classroom evaluation form (cont.)**

6. Did the instructor show respect for the participants?
　　　　__Excellent　__Very good　__Good　　__Fair　__Poor　　__N/A

7. Were the handouts useful?
　　　　__Excellent　__Very good　__Good　　__Fair　__Poor　　__N/A

8. Were you able to read the handouts without difficulty?
　　　　__Excellent　__Very good　__Good　　__Fair　__Poor　　__N/A

9. Were the audio visuals useful?
　　　　__Excellent　__Very good　__Good　　__Fair　__Poor　　__N/A

10. Was the temperature of the classroom comfortable?
　　　　__Excellent　__Very good　__Good　　__Fair　__Poor　　__N/A

11. Were the seating arrangements comfortable?
　　　　__Excellent　__Very good　__Good　　__Fair　__Poor　　__N/A

12. Were you able to see and hear the instructor without difficulty?
　　　　__Excellent　__Very good　__Good　　__Fair　__Poor　　__N/A

13. Were you able to see and hear the A/Vs used without difficulty?
　　　　__Excellent　__Very good　__Good　　__Fair　__Poor　　__N/A

14. Would you like to make any other comments?
_____
_____

15. For future program planning purposes, please identify three specific education topics that would improve your ability to do your job.
_____
_____
_____

16. What would be the easiest, most efficient way for you to attend programs focusing on the topics you identified in #15 above?

Classroom ❑　　　　　　　　　　Audioconference ❑
Self-learning modules ❑　　　　　Computer-based learning ❑
Video or DVD ❑

Other: (Please identify)
_____
_____
_____

EVIDENCE-BASED STAFF DEVELOPMENT

Figure 5.2   **Distance learning evaluation form**

Date: _____

Time: _____

Name (optional): _____

Profession: _____

Department/unit: _____

Program title: _____

Instructor(s): _____

Teaching method: (Please check all that apply)
___Computer-based learning ___Video ___Self-learning packet ___Audiotape___Teleconference

Objectives:
1.
2.
3.

Please answer the following questions: (Note: N/A stands for not applicable)

1. How well did the program content meet the stated objectives?
    __Excellent __Very good __Good __Fair __Poor __N/A

2. Based on the program content, how well were you able to achieve the objectives?
    a. Objective # 1_____
        __Excellent __Very good __Good __Fair __Poor __N/A

    b. Objective #2_____
        __Excellent __Very good __Good __Fair __Poor __N/A

    c. Objective #3_____
        __Excellent __Very good __Good __Fair __Poor __N/A

3. Was the teaching method effective?
    __Excellent __Very good __Good __Fair __Poor __N/A

4. How well were you able to use the equipment for this distance learning experience?
    __Excellent __Very good __Good __Fair __Poor __N/A

5. How well did the program explain how to receive help or to ask questions if you need to do so?

__Excellent __Very good __Good __Fair __Poor __N/A

6. Were the handouts useful?

__Excellent __Very good __Good __Fair __Poor __N/A

7. Were you able to read the handouts without difficulty?

__Excellent __Very good __Good __Fair __Poor __N/A

8. Was the location of this distance learning experience comfortable? In other words, was it quiet and comfortable?

__Excellent __Very good __Good __Fair __Poor __N/A

9. Did the quality of the graphics, videos, or audiotapes help you to learn?

__Excellent __Very good __Good __Fair __Poor __N/A

10. Would you like to make any other comments?

_____
_____
_____
_____

11. For future program planning, please identify three specific education topics that would improve your ability to do your job.

_____
_____
_____
_____

12. What would be the easiest, most efficient way for you to attend programs focusing on the topics you identified in #11 above?

❏ Classroom

❏ Self-learning modules

❏ Video or DVD

❏ Audioconference

❏ Computer-based learning

❏ Other: (Please identify)

who attended Dr. Mason's classes. Preliminary data indicate that patients' responses to chemotherapy are better when the drugs are administered by participants in Dr. Bowman's class.

This scenario shows that education effectiveness does not necessarily depend on the participants' perceptions of the presenter. Further investigation shows that Dr. Bowman spends more time answering questions than does Dr. Mason. Proper data analysis allows the staff development specialist to provide evidence, not opinion or reaction. Evidence indicates that both physicians have particular strengths as presenters, but that Dr. Bowman's educational efforts are more effective. Using objective evidence, Amy is able to work with Dr. Mason and Dr. Bowman to improve the educational experience.

EBP TIP *The key concept here is evidence. Evidence cannot be obtained unless all applicable data are analyzed.*

Analyzing knowledge-acquisition data

Knowledge acquisition is also referred to as learning. To provide evidence that learning has occurred as a result of education, level of knowledge must be assessed prior to and following education. "Simple knowledge acquisition is measured via a pre- and posttest, or appraisal of skill proficiency before and after training" (Avillion 2005).

A comparison of pre- and posttest scores or assessment of skill proficiency before and after training is an objective way to assess knowledge acquisition. Evidence of learning exists only if objective data are available showing an improvement in test scores or in skill proficiency. Again, the word "evidence" triggers the need for an in-depth, objective analysis.

Pre- and posttests and pre– and post–skill assessments have other advantages. Consider this orientation situation:

Orientation to the cardiac care unit requires completion of an educational experience dealing with accurate rhythm strip interpretation and taking appropriate action based on professional standards, licensure, and organizational policies and procedures. Jeremy is the staff development specialist responsible for orientation to the cardiac care unit. He has developed excellent pre- and posttests as well as skill demonstration labs where nurses can demonstrate their ability to intervene in the event of particular arrhythmias.

Five nurses are orienting to the unit. Four of the nurses are new to cardiac care and have no experience in any critical care specialty. The fifth nurse, Lauren, has five years' experience as a cardiac care nurse and is new to this organization. Lauren complains that she is wasting a great deal of time sitting in class and participating in clinical labs, listening to information that she knows quite well. What are some alternatives for Jeremy to take?

Nurses new to the critical care arena may begin orientation with little knowledge of arrhythmias or necessary interventions. However, experienced critical care nurses new to the organization may have extensive knowledge of these issues. It may very well be a waste of an experienced nurse's time to participate in these types of educational programs, but there must be evidence that he or she has the necessary knowledge before participation is deemed unnecessary.

Why not ask Lauren to take the posttest prior to attending class? You can also ask Lauren to demonstrate satisfactory ability to deal with these arrhythmias in the skills lab. If she passes the posttest and demonstrates satisfactory skill performance, there is no need for her to participate in this facet of orientation. The evidence required from all orientees is successful completion of a posttest and successful skill demonstration. Allowing experienced nurses to challenge certain components of orientation will facilitate a more rapid completion of orientation, which will please the orientee, his or her nurse manager, and his or her colleagues.

EBP TIP *In the previous scenario, Lauren demonstrated competency in certain skills and a particular knowledge base. Use this type of EBP to consider making orientation and competency assessment more efficient.*

Analyzing behavior data

Evaluating a learner's behavior requires evidence that he or she is actually applying new knowledge and skills during the performance of job-related duties. Behavior may be evaluated by direct observation, documentation review, and assessment of the appropriateness of patient care interventions (Avillion 2005).

Regardless of the method of assessment, evaluation must be performed consistently. Figure 5.3 is a template for consistent evaluation of behavior.

Evaluators must measure behavior using specific guidelines. You will not be able to use the word "evidence" until all evaluators measure behavior in the same way and according to the same criteria. Additionally, documentation must be objective, and the use of a template is highly

Figure 5.3 — Evaluation of behavior

Date: _____

Time: _____

Objectives:

_____
_____
_____

Evaluation

Medical record review:

_____
_____
_____
_____

Use of equipment:

_____
_____
_____
_____

Direct observation:

_____
_____
_____
_____

Evaluator's comments:

_____
_____
_____
_____
_____

Evaluator's signature:

_____

recommended to ensure consistency. Evaluators should receive training in the evaluation process and use of the template.

These measures are an absolute must. Peer review is becoming more and more common, and ANCC Magnet Recognition Program® surveyors will look for evidence of peer review. It is difficult for friends to evaluate each other's performance objectively—they may be tempted to overlook certain performance problems rather than criticize a friend's behavior. Likewise, two individuals who dislike each other may be tempted to be overly critical when conducting evaluations. As much as possible, avoid asking close friends (and those who are definitely not friends) to evaluate each other.

> **EBP TIP** *When developing templates, make them as objective as possible with space for objectives and expected behaviors. During evaluator training, be sure to stress the need for objectivity and consistency. Explain the importance of obtaining evidence, not opinion.*

Analyzing results data

Even more critical than application of knowledge is the assessment of whether or not education has an impact on job performance and patient outcomes. Here are some kinds of evidence you can look for and document:

- Enhanced patient outcomes (e.g., discharge at a higher level of functioning as measured on an activities of daily living scale following education regarding stroke patient rehabilitation)

- Decrease in the rate of nosocomial infections (e.g., following extensive infection control education)

- Decreased number of patient/family complaints (e.g., following sensitivity training)

Obviously, it takes time to gather these types of data and conduct analysis. It is, in fact, simple research, but it is the only way to provide evidence instead of opinion.

> **EBP TIP** *Be sure to include staff nurses and other healthcare professionals in this type of data collection and analysis. This will give them a feeling of ownership of the project and its success. You may even be able to publish your findings. And don't forget, these types of actions are a plus when applying for Magnet status.*

Think about gathering and analyzing results data in the following situation:

> *Greta is the nurse manager of a 42-bed surgical unit. The length of stay for most patients is about four days. The nurses are responsible for a great deal of patient education prior to discharge, and the unit is always very busy. During the past six months, patient complaints have increased from 10% to 40%. Most of the complaints focus on concerns that the nurses are "rude," "in too much of a hurry to answer questions," and "don't care about the patient's feelings." Greta consults Allison, the staff development specialist responsible for education on the unit, about providing "some type of education" to solve this problem. How should Allison proceed?*

This type of situation is an excellent example of the importance of EBP. The first step Allison should take is to gather evidence to determine if this is a systems problem or an education (lack of knowledge) problem. Working together, Allison, Greta, and the staff RNs determine the following:

- Staff patterns have not changed during the past six months
- The unit has been fully staffed (i.e., no vacancies) for the past eight months
- Patient acuity has remained stable during the past six months
- Roles and responsibilities have remained the same during the past six months

Based on these data, it is determined that external factors are not responsible for attitude change on the unit. During discussions, the RNs made these comments:

- "We're always in a hurry. I guess I don't worry too much about what patients think about me personally, as long as they get good care."

- "It's sad. They [the patients] don't complain about the care they get. But they are upset anyway."

- "How can they think we're rude? They go home better than when they came in."

Allison develops a program that concentrates on sensitivity training and communication skills. She stresses ways for the nurses to give a more positive impression in the time they have available. Some strategies include maintaining eye contact, smiling, greeting the patients by name, and, if they can't stop to answer a nonurgent question immediately, explaining why (briefly and without complaining) and when they will return.

All staff members on the unit, not just the nurses, attend this continuing education program. After everyone has attended and successfully completed the program, patient complaints are analyzed. The percentage of complaints citing rude behavior has gone from 40% to 5% over a six-month period.

This example shows the importance of gathering evidence to analyze possible causes of the problem and following up after program completion to determine if there were actual positive results linked to education.

Analyzing return on investment data

ROI provides evidence that education has had an impact on the organization's financial bottom line (Avillion 2005). This requires the most extensive amount of time of all evaluation types and should be calculated only for programs that have a significant financial impact.

ROI is presented in terms of a percentage. It is calculated by dividing the net program benefits by the program costs and multiplying this answer by 100.

$$ROI\ (\%) = \frac{\text{Net program benefits}}{\text{Program costs}} \times 100$$

You are looking for evidence that the benefits outweigh the costs associated with increasing knowledge acquisition, knowledge application, and positive impact on patient outcomes (i.e., results). Again, objective evidence is the goal. If costs outweigh the benefits, use all available data to make revisions that will increase cost effectiveness without compromising positive impact.

Case study: Assimilation of EBP in staff development

This final case study is a chance for you to use your EBP skills in a challenging situation. Throughout this book, the emphasis has been on transforming your practice and your thinking so that evidence is the foundation of both. EBP in staff development is enhanced when staff development specialists cooperate not only with each other and colleagues from other disciplines within their organization, but when cooperation occurs with those from outside the organization. Gathering evidence, identifying benchmarks, and conducting research are easier and often more productive when data are available from a variety of sources.

Expertise shared among staff development specialists can only increase the body of knowledge that makes the specialty unique. However, collaboration is not always easy, nor is it always effective. Many obstacles exist that cause significant problems. These barriers can even outweigh the advantages of collaboration. Consider the following scenario in which three staff development specialists (from three different organizations) attempt to collaborate on an EBP project they hope will benefit all three of their work settings.

Mike, Nora, and Pilar are staff development specialists who have been friends since earning their bachelor's degrees in nursing 15 years ago. They work at different organizations located about 50 miles apart in rural communities in the mid-western portion of the United States. The three friends meet once a month for lunch. At a recent gathering they were discussing their transitions to EBP in staff development and discovered they had a mutual concern that has triggered a new project at each of their facilities.

All three organizations are about the same size and serve similar populations. Mike, Nora, and Pilar are in the process of developing an ongoing series of programs that deal with various treatment options following myocardial infarction. These staff development specialists have gathered evidence that supports the need for this type of program. They discuss various teaching/learning strategies and are unsure which would be the most effective.

Nora suggests that they collaborate on a research project to identify the most effective method of program delivery. The plan will develop three program options, including classroom style, distance learning, and a blended learning option consisting of both classroom and distance learning. The program objectives are the same for all three options. The three friends will combine resources and ensure consistency of content. They plan to determine the costs of each method and measure program effectiveness using post tests, direct observation in the work setting, and patient outcomes. Mike will deliver the program solely in the classroom setting, Nora will use only distance learning, and Pilar will use a blended learning approach. They hope to be able to publish their project and share their collaborative efforts with staff development specialists on a national level. Since they will be sharing resources, expertise, and outcomes, Mike, Nora, and Pilar approach their managers for approval of a project they feel will be of great benefit to their respective organizations.

Nora and Pilar receive approval and support from their managers. However, Mike does not. His organization's administrative team strongly disapproves of sharing information with the "competition."

What are the options for these three staff development specialists? How would you proceed in these circumstances?

Let's start by looking at what should be considered when proposing a collaborative effort like this one. There are many issues to be addressed in the planning stages.

Prior to attempting collaboration, each staff development specialist should assess the likelihood of receiving support and cooperation from his or her respective facility. Fear of sharing sensitive data and opposition to working with perceived or real competitors are very real concerns. Get to know as much as possible about your organization's philosophy concerning joint projects with other facilities. If you work in a multi-facility organization, you may be able to develop projects by working with staff development professionals from other facilities within your parent organization. Some of these may even be at significant geographic distances from each other, thereby decreasing the competitive dilemma, which exists even within the same organization.

Are the various work settings similar enough in patient care delivery, patient care needs, and staff population to make the outcomes reliable? In other words, treatment options at a major metropolitan hospital may be quite different from those at a small community hospital that transfers patients with complex needs to larger facilities. In the case of Mike, Nora, and Pilar, it must be determined if their organizations are similar enough to warrant identical programs with identical desired outcomes.

 EVIDENCE-BASED STAFF DEVELOPMENT

A written agreement specifying the responsibilities of each staff development specialist is recommended. Issues to address include confidentiality, sharing of expenses, sharing of outcome data, and any potential publishing arrangements.

How will project participants meet? Traveling to a common meeting place is most likely too expensive and time-consuming. Can arrangements be made to do the majority of planning via conference calls, e-mails, and other distance communication methods?

Is it worthwhile for someone in Mike's situation to fight the administrative decision to oppose this project? When proposing this type of project, it is wise to prepare a written proposal that outlines identified expenses, barriers, and potential benefits. A format similar to Figure 4.1 may be helpful, with the potential benefits listed in the evaluation data column. Administrative and management personnel need concise data when deciding whether or not to approve a project. In Mike's situation, continued pressure for approval may even jeopardize Mike's job security. If this refusal to participate is indicative of significant barriers to staff development practice, Mike may even choose to look for another job. Only he can decide if the disadvantages outweigh the advantages of employment with a particular organization.

Program development must also be considered. If, as in this case, a third party cannot participate, the remaining staff development specialists must decide how best to redesign the project. Based on work setting and staffing, Nora and Pilar may choose to work with two methods, distance learning and blended learning, and eliminate the classroom-only method. This decision would be based on program costs, the ability of nurses to leave their work settings to attend a series of classroom programs, etc. Data analysis indicates that classroom setting is the most expensive and least likely to attract an adequate number of participants.

It is imperative that program content be consistent, or outcomes can not be compared. To acquire valid and reliable evidence, Nora and Pilar must make sure that not only is content identical, but that pre- and posttests, distance learning materials, and handouts are the same. Needless to say, objectives and measurement of objective achievement must also be identical.

Nora and Pilar must determine how many nurses should attend the program to obtain an adequate sample size. If the organizations are similar in size, it would be wise to have the same number of participants from each facility.

It is essential that application in the work setting and impact on patient outcomes be measured in the same way. It is easy to develop a pre- and posttest that measures knowledge acquisition. How will application in the work setting be assessed? By direct observation? By evaluating nursing documentation? Figure 5.3 provides an example of a tool that can be used to measure behavior in the work setting with consistency. Failure to be consistent when measuring application in the work setting will significantly compromise findings.

Impact on patient outcomes must also be determined with consistency. What outcomes will be measured and how will they be measured? Length of stay, status at discharge, and ability to perform specific activities of daily living are all examples of patient outcomes.

After implementing the program and analyzing results, Nora and Pilar are able to determine which program was more effective. Effectiveness is measured not only in terms of behavior in the work setting and patient outcomes but on cost of program development and implementation, ease with which participants completed the program, and reactive data. (Note that the same tool should also be used to measure participant reactions to the program.) An evidence-based project such as this enables Nora and Pilar to combine resources to determine program effectiveness based on evidence. They are also able to develop and implement programs in a cost-effective, time-efficient manner by working together and pooling resources. Consider collaboration as part of your EBP.

Reference

Avillion, A. E. (2005). *Nurse Educator Manual: Essential Skills and Guidelines for Effective Practice*. Marblehead, MA: HCPro.

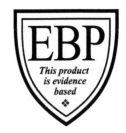

EBP
This product
is evidence
based

Evidence-based staff development practice and predictions for the future

Evidence-based staff development practice and predictions for the future

Learning objectives

After reading this chapter, the participant will be able to:

- Discuss future possibilities for staff development practice

The future of staff development

What does the future hold for staff development specialists? We have seen staff development practice move from informal instruction conducted by nurse managers during the early part of the 20th century to a viable specialty essential to organizational functioning. But this evolution was not easy, and it continues to be a challenge to prove our value in the face of budget cuts and rising healthcare costs.

Predictions cannot be made with complete accuracy, but we can learn from our history to prepare for our future. Here are some predictions for the future of staff development.

1. The need for evidence as a foundation for staff development practice will continue to grow in importance

The premise of this book has been that staff development, like any other healthcare specialty, must conduct business based on evidence of what works, what doesn't, and what should be done to improve services. This includes measuring education's impact on patient outcomes and the financial bottom line.

Indeed, evidence-based practice (EBP) in the clinical arena is an accepted necessity. The financial officers of the organization have always depended on the evidence of facts and figures to determine fiscal solvency. Why is staff development generally behind other departments in areas of fact-based measurement? The struggle to conduct program evaluations that measure impact and ROI continues even today. There are still some staff development specialists who resist these types of evaluations, citing lack of time or fear of having to acknowledge weaknesses in practice.

EBP is another example of staff development failing to be on the cutting edge of specialty practice. We are expected to facilitate EBP of clinicians but fail to promote this concept for ourselves.

Staff development specialists must be innovators when it comes to measuring success, not followers. We need to look to leaders in the field of staff development to help chart our course. But how many of us can quickly identify such leaders? If we don't know them, it may be time to search for them. It may be time for you to become one.

2. EBP requires that more staff development specialists pursue graduate education and develop familiarity with the research process

All levels of staff development specialists can participate in research. However, those who pursue graduate education, particularly at the doctoral level, will be able to facilitate the research process and help others to do so as well. Graduate credentials will also add credibility to the specialty and the findings identified from research.

Think about other healthcare specialties. The entry level for physical therapists may soon be a master's degree. Leaders in other specialties are expected, if not required, to hold graduate degrees.

Thanks to distance learning, it is possible to pursue graduate education from the comfort of your home, sitting at your own computer. It's likely that entry-level education for staff development specialists will soon be at the master's level. We will still utilize all levels of staff in the education process, but the leaders of the field will eventually need graduate preparation.

3. Accreditation organizations will expect that all departments within the organization function based on EBP

The Joint Commission and ANCC Magnet Recognition Program® surveyors are looking for evidence that all members of an organization work together to facilitate quality patient outcomes. This includes evaluating current practice, identifying strengths and weaknesses, and developing processes to continually monitor and improve services. How can this take place unless there is an objective system of gathering and analyzing data to document evidence? EBP is not only a logical means of improving products and services; it is also a means of being in constant readiness for unannounced surveys by accreditation surveyors.

4. Competency of staff development specialists will need to be formally assessed and documented

Brunt (2007) identifies several applications of staff development competencies. These applications will enhance staff development practice.

Staff development competencies:

- Can serve as a balanced approach for graduate education in the field of staff development

- Can help gather evidence for the revision of The American Nurses Association's *Scope and Standards of Practice for Nursing Professional Development*

- Can serve as a resource for the nursing professional development certification exam prepared by the American Nurses Credentialing Center

- Can serve as evidence when assessing job performance and developing job descriptions

- Can serve as the foundation of orienting persons to the role of staff development specialist

- Can serve as a guide for professional staff development practice and documentation of the role "Nurses as Teachers," one of the Forces of Magnetism

Conclusion

No one can predict the future with 100% accuracy, but study the evolution of staff development as a guide to preparing yourself for your future as a staff development specialist. EBP will serve as a strong foundation for you and your department, and will provide evidence of your value to the organization.

Change and challenge are part of every professional's world. But, by implementing EBP, you will be ready to deal with both.

Reference

Brunt, B. (2007). *Competencies for Staff Educators: Tools to Evaluate and Enhance Nursing Professional Development.* Marblehead, MA: HCPro.

Nursing education
instructional guide

Nursing education instructional guide

Evidence-Based Staff Development: Strategies to Create, Measure, and Refine Your Program

Target audience

Directors of Education

Staff Development Specialists

Directors of Nursing

VPs of Nursing

Chief Nursing Officers

Nurse Managers

HR Directors

Statement of need

Evidence-based practice (EBP) is the buzz in nursing, and staff development specialists are expected to facilitate this practice among their clinical customers. This book takes EBP guidelines and applies them to staff development practice. It is a practical guide to help staff development specialists develop their services in ways that provide evidence about how their services impact the organization and how they use objective evidence to revise their services. With today's emphasis on cost-containment and accountability, it is critical that educators measure their effectiveness and demonstrate their value to the organization. This book guides staff educators through gathering evidence to evaluate the current effectiveness of their staff development practice, and gives them the information they need to use consistent, objective, validated tools to assist them as they improve their departments. (This activity is intended for individual use only.)

Educational objectives

Upon completion of this activity, participants should be able to:

- Explain the use of evidence in staff development practice
- Review sources for gathering data/evidence for staff development practice
- Summarize the historical issues that contribute to evidence-based staff development practice
- Discuss the advantages and barriers to EBP in staff development
- Explain the ethical implications of EBP in staff development
- Identify legal implications of EBP in staff development
- Explain how to acquire support from staff, management, and administration for the implementation of EBP in staff development
- Formulate strategies for the implementation of EBP in staff development
- Explain how EBP in staff development helps to achieve and maintain Magnet® status
- Apply program evaluation data to EBP in staff development
- Discuss future possibilities for staff development practice

Faculty

Adrianne E. Avillion, D.Ed., RN, is the owner of Avillion's Curriculum Design in York, PA. A past president of the National Nursing Staff Development Organization (NNSDO), she specializes in freelance medical writing and designing continuing education programs for healthcare professionals. She also offers consulting services in work redesign, quality improvement, and staff development.

Avillion has published extensively, including serving as editor of the first and second editions of *The Core Curriculum for Staff Development,* published by NNSDO. Her most recent publications include *A Practical Guide to Staff Development: Tools and Techniques for Effective Education,* published by HCPro, Inc. and *Nurse Entrepreneurship: The Art of Running Your Own Business,* published by Creative Health Care Management. She is also a frequent presenter at conferences and conventions devoted to the specialty of continuing education and staff development.

 EVIDENCE-BASED STAFF DEVELOPMENT

Accreditation/Designation statement

HCPro is accredited as a provider of continuing nursing education by the American Nurses Credentialing Center Commission on Accreditation.

This educational activity for three nursing contact hours is provided by HCPro, Inc.

Faculty disclosure statement

HCPro, Inc., has confirmed that none of the faculty/presenters or contributors have any relevant financial relationships to disclose related to the content of this educational activity.

Instructions

In order to be eligible to receive your nursing contact hours for this activity, you are required to do the following:

1. Read the book *Evidence-Based Staff Development: Strategies to Create, Measure, and Refine Your Program*
2. Complete the exam
3. Complete the evaluation
4. Provide your contact information on the exam and evaluation
5. Submit your exam and evaluation to HCPro, Inc.

Please provide all of the information requested above and mail or fax your completed exam, program evaluation, and contact information to:

HCPro, Inc.
Attn: Continuing Education Department
200 Hoods Lane
Marblehead, MA 01945
Fax: 781/639-2982

NOTE:

This book and associated exam are intended for individual use only. If you would like to provide this continuing education exam to other members of your nursing staff, please contact our customer service department at 877/727-1728 to place your order. The exam fee schedule is as follows:

Exam quantity	Fee
1	$0
2–25	$15 per person
26–50	$12 per person
51–100	$8 per person
101+	$5 per person

EVIDENCE-BASED STAFF DEVELOPMENT

Continuing education exam

Name: _____

Title: _____

Facility name: _____

Address: _____

Address: _____

City: _____ State: _____ ZIP: _____

Phone number: _____ Fax number: _____

E-mail: _____

Nursing license number: _____

(ANCC requires a unique identifier for each learner.)

Date completed: _____

1. The implementation of evidence-based staff development practice:

    a. Has little or no impact on patient outcomes

    b. Is swiftly implemented thanks to the abundant amount of staff development research data

    c. Should enhance job performance

    d. Is well understood by most staff development specialists

2. A staff development specialist who has some experience in the specialty but has trouble prioritizing tasks and dealing with unexpected situations is most likely:

    a. A novice

    b. An advanced beginner

    c. Competent

    d. Proficient

3. A proficient staff development specialist:

    a. Depends on rules and guidelines to guide his or her performance

    b. Has no prior experience in staff development

    c. Lacks speed and proficiency

    d. Instinctively views a situation as a whole rather than as individual aspects

4. Amy is a pediatric clinical nurse specialist. During her 15 years as a registered nurse she has worked exclusively as a pediatric clinician. Amy is considering entering the staff development field. As a staff development specialist, she would be considered:

    a. A novice

    b. An expert

    c. Proficient

    d. Competent

5. Evidence-based clinical practice:

    a. Relies on research studies conducted at specific internals

    b. Helps practitioners to close the gap between actual and best practice

    c. Has no direct correlation to evidence-based staff development practice

    d. Is geared to those nurses who are doctorally prepared and trained in research

6. Data for evidence-based staff development practice:

    a. Should be obtained solely from educational program evaluations

    b. Are useful only if gathered from formal research studies

    c. Are used to bridge the gap between actual staff development practice and best practices in staff development

    d. Are discounted if obtained from nonclinical sources

7. Which of the following statements about gathering data for EBP in staff development is accurate?

    a. Competency statements should correlate with staff development products and services

    b. Data from performance evaluations is confidential and cannot be used as evidence in program planning

    c. Organizational goals are too broad to impact staff development planning and implementation

    d. Informal conversations with staff are not reliable sources of data

8. All of the following statements about competency-based education (CBE) are true EXCEPT:

    a. CBE correlates with research and EBP

    b. CBE focuses on outcomes

    c. CBE gained prominence during the 1960s

    d. CBE is an educator-centered philosophy

EVIDENCE-BASED STAFF DEVELOPMENT

9. Nursing research:

 a. Dates at least from the 1960s

 b. Is valid and reliable only if conducted by doctorally prepared researchers

 c. Includes the documentation of findings to facilitate implementation

 d. Is not necessary if a nurse's instincts tell him or her how to identify the best intervention

10. The top source of information on which nurses rely for evidence regarding their practice is:

 a. Experience

 b. Intuition

 c. Past usual practice

 d. Workplace sources

11. Historical events have had great impact on the specialty of staff development. Which of these statements is accurate regarding the evolution of the specialty?

 a. The need for a distinct department devoted to the continuing education of nurses was mandated during the Great Depression

 b. The first credentialing exam for nursing continuing education and professional development was offered in the 1970s

 c. World War II triggered a need for an increase in the number of nonprofessional healthcare providers

 d. Florence Nightingale was responsible for the establishment of the first staff development department within the hospital setting

12. EBP in staff development can lead to all of the following EXCEPT:

 a. Enhanced communication among departments

 b. Stimulation of interest in the research process

 c. Widening of the gap between theory and practice

 d. Improving the cost-effectiveness of educational offerings

13. Resistance to EBP in staff development:

 a. Is unlikely to come from staff development specialists

 b. Is not a significant barrier to its implementation

 c. Can be viewed as an advantage because resistance requires careful opposition

 d. Can come from other departments as well as administration

14. **It is reasonable to expect that implementation of staff development EBP:**

   a. Requires significant time to gather and analyze data

   b. Is the responsibility of the staff development manager and will not affect other members of the staff development department

   c. Will not require additional financial resources

   d. May necessitate that all staff development specialists be doctorally prepared

15. **Ethical dilemmas are:**

   a. Usually swiftly resolved because there is generally one easy solution

   b. The result of conflicting moral claims

   c. Based on two sets of values: one that is right and one that is wrong

   d. Triggered by resistance to administrative directives

16. **Wrongful conduct, failure to properly discharge professional duties, or failure to meet standards of care that result in harm to another person is:**

   a. Negligence

   b. Breach of duty

   c. Malpractice

   d. Liability

17. **Legal responsibility for the failure to act or taking action that does not meet standards of care thus causing harm to another person is called:**

   a. Liability

   b. Malpractice

   c. Negligence

   d. Duty

18. **Staff development specialists may be somewhat resistant to the implementation of change. All of the following are normal facets of resistance EXCEPT:**

   a. Fear of failure

   b. Sabotage

   c. Questioning

   d. Anxiety about new responsibilities

EVIDENCE-BASED STAFF DEVELOPMENT

19. When conducting the initial meeting regarding implementation of EBP with your staff development specialists, you should:

    a. Complete an action plan prior to the conclusion of the meeting

    b. Avoid discussing barriers to its implementation

    c. Address fears and concerns honestly

    d. Establish implementation goals and present them to your staff

20. When discussing the implementation of staff development EBP with administration, it is important to:

    a. Ask for an increase in the amount of money in the staff development budget

    b. Explain that EBP will not affect how your department communicates with the rest of the organization

    c. Ask for additional staff development positions

    d. Describe how EBP will facilitate accreditation achievement

21. Identification of best practices:

    a. Can be made after reviewing data from a one-time program presentation

    b. Is not associated with EBP

    c. Is determined as part of data analysis

    d. Must be determined by management

22. Benchmarks are:

    a. Validated by a history of best practices

    b. Identified by administration

    c. Not applicable in the staff development setting

    d. Formulated quickly

23. All of the following statements concerning the implementation of EBP in staff development are accurate EXCEPT:

    a. Successful implementation of EBP depends on the cooperation of all staff development specialists within the organization

    b. Ongoing data analysis is essential to EBP

    c. Benchmarks are hypothetical concepts that cannot be identified via EBP

    d. Identification of best practices is part of the EBP process

24. The Magnet Force of autonomy relies on staff development services to:

   a. Dictate what nurses may or may not do as part of their practice

   b. Provide education that helps nurses move from novice to expert

   c. Conduct research that highlights flaws in nursing practice

   d. Discourage independent judgment for fear of malpractice actions

25. Staff development's role in the community presence of the organization:

   a. Has little or no impact on Magnet recognition

   b. Should not involve patient education since that is primarily the responsibility of the staff nurse

   c. Involves the opportunity for collaborative research concerning patient outcomes following
      patient education

   d. Relies on receiving a request from administration to participate in community efforts

26. The role of teacher in the Magnet process:

   a. Is limited to staff development specialists

   b. Requires that only nurses with graduate education function as teachers

   c. Relies on the staff development specialist to educate staff nurses in the teaching/learning process

   d. Is limited to the inpatient setting

27. Resources to maintain competency are part of the staff development role in which Magnet force?

   a. Professional development

   b. Leadership

   c. Image of nursing

   d. Autonomy

28. Which of the following statements is a description of reactive data?

   a. Patient falls have decreased by 15%

   b. There was a 10% profit from a patient safety program

   c. 40% of participants felt that the instructor did not allow enough time for discussion

   d. 100% of the participants achieved passing scores on a posttest

29. A Magnet surveyor is looking for evidence that a spinal cord injury (SCI) continuing education
program had a positive impact on patient outcomes. She would be pleased to find that after nurses
participated in this program:

EVIDENCE-BASED STAFF DEVELOPMENT

a. Their nurse manager believed that job satisfaction increased

b. There was an increase in the number of nurses hired to work on the SCI unit

c. 100% of the participants achieved a passing score on a test assessing knowledge of SCI

d. There was a 20% increase in the number of patients able to function independently at discharge

30. **90% of nurses who participated in a distance learning program stated that they preferred to attend classroom education activities. The staff development specialist responsible for implementing that program should:**

a. Analyze data concerning application of knowledge and patient outcomes

b. Convert the program to a classroom activity

c. Discount the data since it is only reactive in nature

d. Realize that this is evidence that the program was ineffective

31. **Evaluation conducted via a pre- and posttest provides evidence of:**

a. Reaction

b. Knowledge acquisition

c. Results

d. ROI

32. **You are interested in determining whether a housewide program's benefits outweigh the costs. You would assess:**

a. Results/impact

b. Learning

c. ROI

d. Reaction

33. **Which of these situations describe adequate application of knowledge?**

a. Monica passes a posttest regarding the pathophysiology of ovarian cancer with a score of 100%

b. David tells the staff development specialist that he really enjoyed the distance learning activity she developed

c. The nurse manager of the oncology unit notes that medication errors have decreased by 10%

d. A preceptor notes that a new nurse correctly administers an injection to a pediatric patient after attending a class on pediatric medications

34. Which of these pieces of evidence shows that education has had an impact on patient outcomes?

a. A nurse correctly draws an arterial blood gas sample after receiving training in the procedure

b. The number of geriatric patients experiencing a compromise in skin integrity decreases by 50% following a program on skin care and nursing interventions for geriatric patients

c. 90% of program participants rate the instructor as extremely knowledgeable

d. The ROI on a patient safety program is 30%

35. Data dealing with learner satisfaction is:

a. Reactive

b. Knowledge acquisition

c. Knowledge application

d. ROI

36. Competencies for staff development specialists:

a. Are not as critical as the need for clinical competencies

b. Have little impact on the pursuit of Magnet status

c. Serve as a balanced approach for graduate education

d. Cannot be identified due to the wide variety of roles of the staff development specialist

37. All of the following statements concerning the future of staff development are accurate EXCEPT:

a. Accreditation organizations will expect all departments to function via EBP

b. The need for EBP in staff development will continue to grow

c. EBP in staff development enhances the pursuit of Magnet status

d. EBP in staff development will decrease the need for staff development competencies

 EVIDENCE-BASED STAFF DEVELOPMENT

Continuing education evaluation

Name: _____

Title: _____

Facility name: _____

Address: _____

Address: _____

City: _____ State: _____ ZIP: _____

Phone number: _____ Fax number: _____

E-mail: _____

Nursing license number: _____

(ANCC requires a unique identifier for each learner.)

Date completed: _____

1. **This activity met the learning objectives stated:**

Strongly Agree   Agree   Disagree   Strongly Disagree

2. **Objectives were related to the overall purpose/goal of the activity:**

Strongly Agree   Agree   Disagree   Strongly Disagree

3. **This activity was related to my continuing education needs:**

Strongly Agree   Agree   Disagree   Strongly Disagree

4. **The exam for the activity was an accurate test of the knowledge gained:**

Strongly Agree   Agree   Disagree   Strongly Disagree

5. **The activity avoided commercial bias or influence:**

Strongly Agree   Agree   Disagree   Strongly Disagree

6. **This activity met my expectations:**

Strongly Agree   Agree   Disagree   Strongly Disagree

7. Will this activity enhance your professional practice?

Yes   No

8. The format was an appropriate method for delivery of the content for this activity:

Strongly Agree   Agree   Disagree   Strongly Disagree

9. If you have any comments on this activity, please note them here:

10. How much time did it take for you to complete this activity?

Thank you for completing this evaluation of our continuing education activity!

Return completed form to:

HCPro, Inc.
Attn: Continuing Education Department
200 Hoods Lane, Marblehead, MA 01945
Tel: 877/727-1728
Fax: 781/639-2982

EVIDENCE-BASED STAFF DEVELOPMENT